THE
SKIN
COMMANDMENTS

THE SKIN

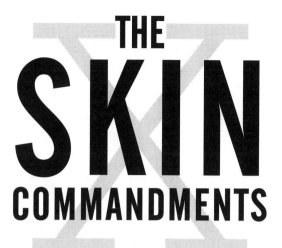

COMMANDMENTS

10 RULES TO HEALTHY,
BEAUTIFUL SKIN

DR. TONY NAKHLA

AMERICA'S DERMATOLOGIST

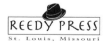
REEDY PRESS
St. Louis, Missouri

Reedy Press
PO Box 5131
St. Louis, MO 63139, USA

Photo Credits:
iStock: 11, 14, 24, 27, 29, 31, 38, 40, 46, 47, 51, 52, 54, 60, 62, 63, 64, 66, 67, 70, 78, 84, 86, 98, 99, 100, 103, 104, 106, 108, 113, 115, 118, 120, 125, 128, 135, 138
OC Skin Institute: 12, 122, 123, 126

Library of Congress Control Number: 2011936120

ISBN: 978-1-935806-06-6

Cover design by Michael Nagin
Interior design by Jill Halpin

Please visit our website at www.reedypress.com.

Printed in the United States of America
11 12 13 14 15   5 4 3 2 1

to Mom

Contents

Acknowledgments

I thank God for the countless blessings in my life and for the opportunities I have been given. Thanks to my mother Tahany, my sisters Jean and Nora, my brothers Mike and Tom, Luke and Mikayla, Dr. Refaat Abraham, Dr. Amgad Girgis, and my entire cast of family and friends.

To my mentor Dr. David C. Horowitz, program director and chair of the Department of Dermatology at Western University of Health Sciences, who ignited and continues to guide me in my career.

A special thanks to my great friend Raymond Garcia at Penguin Group-USA for his encouragement and efforts in launching this project and tremendous input throughout the production. To the team at Reedy Press, Josh Stevens and Matt Heidenry, for believing in this book concept and seeing it through. To Patricia Corrigan for her literary expertise, insightful editing, and amazing work. To Liam Collopy, Shannon Donnelly, and the entire team at Levine Communications for their world-class publicity efforts. To Dr. Andrew Abraham, Marco Borges, Dr. Craig Ziering, and Dr. David Matlock for their kind words and support.

I am sincerely grateful.

THE SKIN COMMANDMENTS

INTRODUCTION

EVERYONE WANTS GREAT SKIN

People all over the world turn to cosmetic products and skin-care treatments to help clear their acne, brighten their complexion, or reduce the signs of aging.

Who do they turn to for skin-care advice?

Cindy Crawford, the Kardashian sisters, P-Diddy, Jessica Simpson, and other celebrities endorse skin-care regimens on infomercials. Beauty counters in every large department store carry "miracle" creams and electronic facial brushes. Interactive websites are standing by to help you determine your skin type and advise you on which products to purchase. Moms and grandmas offer their own home remedies as well.

Who best can help you make good choices, based on expert opinion instead of celebrity status, million-dollar marketing campaigns, computer-generated algorithms, or old wives' tales?

I can.

I'm Dr. Tony Nakhla, a board-certified dermatologist, skin cancer surgeon, cosmetic surgeon, and an osteopathic physician with extensive training in both traditional and holistic medicine as well as nutrition.

As an expert in multiple, often-conflicting fields, in *The Skin Commandments* I capture the tremendous synergy of modern treatments, holistic principles, and nature-based regimens. I help you understand how all of these methods can be successfully employed in the optimal care of your skin.

For instance: _____

- Botox and pomegranate make a dynamic duo in reversing signs of aging.
- Green tea goes well with a laser treatment or chemical peel.
- Coconut water complements topical moisturizers.

In this book, I also answer many common skin-care questions, including: _____

- How does drinking water affect my skin?
- Which foods can improve my complexion?
- What cleansers and moisturizers should I use?
- Are tanning beds safer than the sun?

These are the kinds of questions and concerns I regularly answer for my patients at OC Skin Institute, my practice in Southern California. My patients include older women who want to reverse the signs of aging, young women who hope to preserve their natural beauty, working moms, models, actors, and Hollywood stars. Many are men who wish to put their best face forward, achieve a youthful look, or restore their confidence.

Like you, all these individuals want to take the best possible care of their skin.

Everything you need to know about caring for your skin is here, presented in ten simple steps, or "commandments," that will help you achieve healthy, beautiful skin.

Commandments I-IV focus on adopting healthy behaviors, proper skin hygiene, and using topical skin-care products. Commandment V covers various methods of exfoliation to give your skin a healthy glow. Commandment VI emphasizes the importance of antioxidants in topical skin-care regimens, in food, and in dietary supplements.

Commandments VII, VIII, and IX cover advanced treatments and procedures that help you fend off or reverse signs of aging. The final Commandment explores how to live a healthy life, one that will help keep your skin healthy, and beautiful, no matter what your age.

At the beginning of each chapter, I briefly outline how to "obey" each Commandment and give the bottom-line instructions. Throughout the book, you will find "breakouts" (that's an intended dermatology pun) that summarize important information, offer fun facts, or enlarge upon the narrative text. Plenty of illustrations and photos are included as well.

Remember, prices for treatments may vary from region to region, so the dollar amounts I provide here are estimates. But if you seek practical information about skin care, if you have questions about anti-aging regimens, if you want to know what it takes to have healthy, glowing skin—this is the book for you.

Before I share with you *The Skin Commandments*, let's talk about skin.

Skin is the largest organ. It covers us and protects us. The skin of an average adult measures about 3,000 square inches and weighs close to six pounds.

Human skin is composed of three layers that play a significant role in health and beauty:

- the epidermis
- the dermis
- the subcutaneous fat

Human Skin:
An Overview

THE EPIDERMIS

The epidermis is the outer layer of skin. Think of an onion with multiple layers of peel. The outermost peeling layer is rough and sheds, while the inner layers are smooth and solid, providing the structure of the onion.

Like the flaky outer layer of an onion, the epidermis also constantly sheds. This outer layer of skin is responsible for texture, including a dry or peeling appearance when skin is not adequately moisturized.

Now think of an onion that is growing from its central core, expanding from the inside out. The more it grows, the more the inner layers move out to the surface, where they eventually become the outermost peeling layer.

This is precisely how human skin acts.

Skin constantly grows from the inside out, shedding old skin cells at the surface. Below the surface, new baby skin cells are produced and the process repeats itself. The more the exfoliation process is helped or enhanced (by creams, chemical peels, lasers, dermabrasion, and other treatments), the smoother and more beautiful the outermost surface of the skin.

These treatments target the epidermis, removing old skin cells at the surface in order to smooth the texture and appearance and get down to deeper layers of brighter, softer, more radiant skin.

THE DERMIS

Below the epidermis lies the dermis. This dense layer is composed mainly of collagen, elastic fibers, and tougher materials that give the skin its stretchable quality, or elasticity.

Think of a rubber band. When you stretch and release a rubber band, it snaps back to its original size. Skin has a similar property. If you tug on it and then release it, your skin returns to its original shape.

The skin's elasticity—its ability to stretch and return to normal shape—is determined by the amount and the strength of elastic fibers within the dermis. Elastic fibers (referred to as elastin in medical terminology) naturally break down and weaken over time due to age and the harmful effects of sunlight, tanning, and oxidative damage from free radicals. (Learn more in Skin Commandment VI: Fight Free Radicals.)

Youthful skin has a high level of elasticity, with strong elastic fibers, which explains why young people have skin that quickly bounces back when stretched, and appears tight and smooth.

In contrast, older skin or sun-damaged skin possess much less elasticity. Often, older skin appears loose and saggy. Sun damage, age, and the effects of gravity are to blame. (Tanning—and the importance of not tanning—is covered in detail in Skin Commandment I: Thou Shalt Not Tan.)

Epidermis

Dermis

Subcutaneous Fat

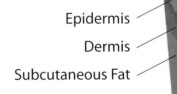

SUBCUTANEOUS FAT

Below the epidermis and the dermis is a viscous, jelly-like material called subcutaneous fat. The amount of subcutaneous fat varies from region to region. There is more in the buttocks, for example, than in the back of the hands.

This subcutaneous fat provides skin with a plump, healthy appearance. Young people have full, round faces, while the skin of elderly people appear thin and translucent, creating what is referred to as a skin-on-bone appearance. This is due to the normal aging process. Over time, the amount of subcutaneous fat in the face and other body parts literally dissolves, resulting in a hollowed-out appearance.

Many injectable cosmetic treatments are available to plump up the skin. In some procedures, subcutaneous fat is moved from one area to another. In others, materials that safely mimic the subcutaneous fat are injected. Other procedures stimulate your body's own collagen to help re-volumize the skin. In all instances, the skin is restored to its original look and texture, and the face appears plump once again. (These products and others are described at length in Skin Commandment VIII: Fill 'er Up.)

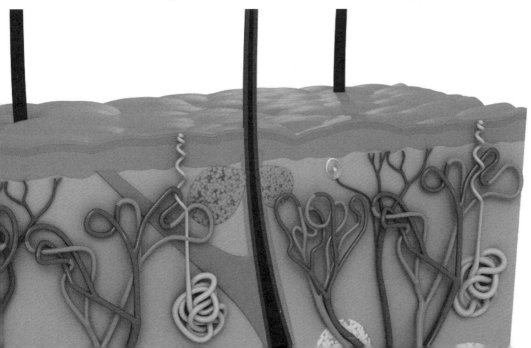

What Lies Below

Below the three layers of skin are muscle, bone, and our internal organs. The skin literally acts as an envelope for the entire human body. Skin is sometimes referred to as a window to the inner body.

Messages from the internal organs are displayed in the form of changes in the physical appearance of the skin. In other words, dysfunctions of the inner organs are frequently visible on the skin's surface, manifesting as rashes or other skin maladies. These signs alert doctors that something is wrong inside the body.

It is important to envision the body as a machine. Like any machine, the longer it runs, the more wear and tear occurs—wear and tear that often is visible on the skin. Over time, damage from sun, wind, free radicals, and pollutants also give skin a weathered, leathery appearance.

Feeling and looking healthy requires a holistic approach and an understanding that when the body is functioning perfectly inside, it gleams with beauty on the outside.

A healthy body manifests healthy skin—and healthy skin is beautiful skin.

With a little help from you, your dermatologist, and *The Skin Commandments*, the possibilities are endless.

Let's get started!

THE SKIN COMMANDMENTS

SKIN
COMMANDMENT
THOU SHALT NOT TAN

OBEYING SKIN COMMANDMENT I

Skin Commandment I is not optional.
Never tan. Ever.

Use sunscreen on your face every day.

If you are outdoors for extended periods of time,
put sunscreen on your face and any sun-exposed areas,
wear a hat, and try to stay in the shade.

Choose a sunscreen with a high sun protection factor (SPF)
and broad-spectrum (both UVA and UVB) protection.

Use bronzer, sunless tanning lotions,
or spray tan as safe alternatives to tanning.

You may not need to read an entire chapter to know tanning is bad for you. If you've already sworn off baking in the sun, you may choose to skip Skin Commandment I, but in this chapter you also will learn:

– how to choose a sunscreen

– how to properly apply sunscreen

– how to check yourself for skin cancer

– how to adopt healthy behaviors outdoors

– interesting skin cancer facts

– how to safely and effectively bronze your skin

Where does a doctor practicing in beach-abundant Southern California get off telling people not to tan, catch some rays, "lay out," bronze up?

Here's where: —————————————————

On a daily basis, my job as a skin cancer surgeon is to remove tumors from patients' faces. Some of those patients are beautiful young women. In many cases, as part of my job I must inform people that they may die from a cancer they could have prevented.

I would be a traitor to my profession if I didn't say at the start of the first chapter of this book that tanning is an unhealthy, unattractive, and dangerous behavior. Lying out in the sun as a way to achieve beautiful skin is like trying to whiten your teeth while drinking coffee or like trying to lower your cholesterol while continuing to eat red meat.

Tanning is counterproductive. Tanning is illogical. If you embrace any skin enhancement or anti-aging program—and even if you do not—when it comes to tanning and excessive sun exposure:

Don't Do It.

The Dark Side
of Tanning

Some people think it's healthy to get some sun and often refer to darkened skin as a "healthy" tan.

These people are terribly mistaken.

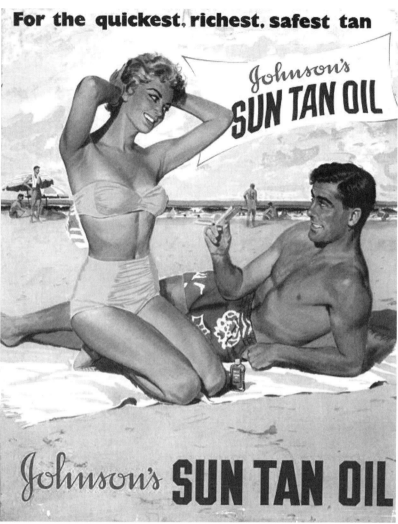

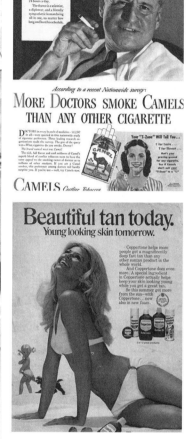

Tanning is to skin what smoking is to the lungs. In the 1940s, smoking and tanning were in vogue, symbols of glamour. Going out with friends meant having a smoke. Going to the beach meant slathering baby oil on your body and baking in the sun. Both harmful habits were considered healthy, and many advertising campaigns echoed that point of view.

Today, the American Heart Association considers cigarette smoking the most important preventable cause of premature death. More than 440,000 people die from smoking-related diseases every year. Fortunately, the rate of smoking has decreased significantly in the past decades due to effective campaigns and educational programs.

Tanning—the most harmful human habit affecting skin—continues to be an accepted part of Western culture and is falsely considered healthy by many. Even popular reality TV shows like *Sunset Tan*, *Real Housewives*, and *The Jersey Shore* have featured hard-body, main characters baking themselves in tanning beds to achieve a better look, one that is considered attractive, even sexy.

In 2010, the National Cancer Institute estimated reports of more than one million new cases of skin cancer in the United States. In sun-worshipping Australia, two-thirds of Aussies will be diagnosed with skin cancer by the time they reach seventy.

Tanning Beds
Are Not the Answer

Here's a bad idea I hear a lot: "I'm going to a huge event tonight and I need to look good, so I'll probably hit the tanning bed beforehand."

Many people are under the impression that tanning beds are a safe alternative to lying out in the sun. Well, they're wrong. The risk of melanoma is nearly 75 percent higher for people who use tanning beds than for those who do not. The Department of Health and Human Services has declared that ultraviolet (UV) rays from the sun and from tanning beds to be known carcinogens—cancer-causing substances.

Yet on an average day, more than one million people show up at tanning salons in the United States, ready to strip down and expose their bodies to cancer-causing rays.

Nearly 70 percent of people who use tanning beds are Caucasian women ages sixteen to twenty-nine. Young women are at the highest risk for melanoma, and we know that exposure to UV light is a risk factor for this deadly cancer.

It's a recipe for disaster. Blame the Food and Drug Administration's lack of regulation and the tanning-bed industry itself, which boasted an estimated $2.6 billion in revenue in 2010.

Yes—tanning, in this day and age, is somehow considered a symbol of health and beauty. The exact opposite is true. Tanning is unhealthy, and its effects are ugly.

Ask What Tanning Can Do for You

– Tanning causes skin cancer.

– Tanning causes wrinkles.

– Tanning causes blotchy sunspots on the skin.

– Tanning makes you look older.

– Tanning—in case you missed it—can kill you.

Burning vs. Tanning

Depending on your complexion and ancestral lineage, your skin may turn bright red after prolonged sun exposure, resulting in sunburn. Others "pink up" first and turn brown later. Others tan without ever turning pink or burning.

Some people tell themselves, "It's okay that I'm sunburned or a little pink right now, it will turn into a tan later, so I'm fine."

These people would be wrong—real wrong.

Sunburn is your skin's way of shouting, "Fire!"

Sunburned skin is damaged skin, and the damage is done much deeper than you might expect. When your skin burns, blisters, and peels, your skin is not happy—or healthy. Plus, just three or four bad sunburns when you are a child put you at an increased risk of melanoma as an adult. Moms and dads, now is a good time to start using sunscreen on your children.

Other people—the people whose skin turns toasty brown—also think they are in no danger because exposure to the sun does not cause them to turn lobster red. "I never burn," these people say, "so the sun can't hurt me."

These people would also be wrong—real wrong.

According to the Centers for Disease Control, melanomas occur in Caucasians 20 percent more often than in African-Americans. That is because there is a genetic predisposition to developing skin cancer and also because the level of pigment in black skin and brown skin provides extra protection from the sun.

That said, individuals with dark-pigmented skin also can develop skin cancer, including melanoma, and when they do, it is even more lethal than in other populations. Bob Marley is one example of a dark-skinned individual who died from melanoma.

Browning your skin is just as dangerous. When you expose your unprotected skin to the sun, your body responds by creating its own sunscreen—called melanin pigment.

Think of tanning as your skin's way of yelling, **"Hey, you forgot to put on sunscreen!"**

Melanin pigment is what gives your skin its tan color. Unfortunately, the production of melanin pigment is slow and does not occur in time to protect you from the sun's harmful rays. As you may recall, your skin becomes tan several hours or days after sun exposure. By that point, the damage is already done.

Over time, after repeated bouts of unprotected sun exposure, your skin becomes unable to regulate the production of this pigment, leaving your skin tone blotchy, as though a pen has exploded and splattered ink all over your purse or pocket.

The Culprit:
The Sun's Ultraviolet Rays

How can something so good at sustaining life on our planet, so proficient at helping crops grow, so effective at lifting our mood, be so bad for our skin?

Ultraviolet rays come from the sun. Tanning beds use artificial UV rays. Both are extremely harmful to the skin. UV rays penetrate the skin and directly affect the DNA of skin cells, causing them to transform over time into cancerous cells.

As I explained in the Introduction, normal skin cells slowly grow from the inside out and then shed at the surface. UV rays disrupt normal cell growth, speed it up, and put skin cells into uncontrollable overdrive. This disorderly, out-of-control skin-cell growth results in skin cancer, which appears as growths or tumors on the surface of the skin. Skin cancer often requires surgery and can result in horrific scars on the face. Skin cancer can also result in death.

Here, from the National Cancer Institute,
are the three most common types of skin cancer:

- Skin cancer that forms in the lower part of the epidermis (the outer layer of the skin) is called basal cell carcinoma.

- Skin cancer that forms in squamous cells (flat cells that form the surface of the skin) is called squamous cell carcinoma.

- Skin cancer that forms in melanocytes (skin cells that make melanin pigment) is called melanoma.

Skin cancer is the most common form of cancer in the United States. Melanoma is one of the most deadly forms of all types of cancer.

Basal cell and squamous cell carcinomas, the two most common types of skin cancer, are highly curable. The treatment, however, usually results in significant scarring.

Melanoma is deadly. The National Cancer Institute estimated more than 68,000 new cases and 8,700 deaths due to melanoma in 2010.

Holy Moley!

"My moles look strange. Could they be cancerous?"

They could.

Every year, more people than ever before are diagnosed with skin cancer. What should you watch for?

- slow-growing pink bumps on your skin that crust over and bleed

- raised wart-like growths that form ulcers

- multi-colored moles with uneven borders or moles that change size, shape, or color

If you spy any of these growing anywhere on your body—and yes, you should check your skin often for these signs—make an appointment with a dermatologist. The American Academy of Dermatology recommends that everyone be examined for skin cancer once a year. Since 1985, the Academy has worked with dermatologists across the United States to offer free skin cancer screenings. To find one near you, see www.aad.org/public/exams/screenings/index.html.

Dr. Darrell S. Rigel and his colleagues from the Department of Dermatology at the New York University School of Medicine offer an easy way to help you identify signs of melanoma. Think A-B-C-D.

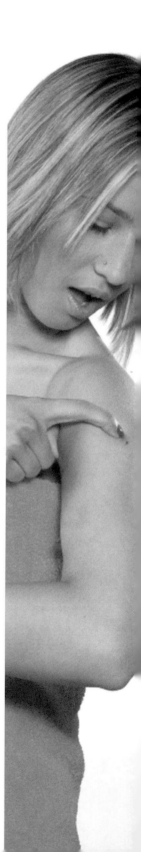

A	B	C	D
is for asymmetry	**is for border**	**is for color**	**is for diameter**
If I draw a line through the center of my mole, are the two halves equal in size and shape (good) or unequal (bad)?	Are the outer borders of my mole smooth (good) or are they jagged (bad)?	Is my mole tan in color (good) or is it a dark black color (bad)? Is my mole one uniform color throughout (good) or does my mole have multiple colors (bad)?	Is my mole smaller than a pencil eraser (good) or bigger (bad)?

Asymmetry

Border Irregularity

Color

1/4 Inch Diameter

Got that? **Good!**

We know that most skin cancers can be prevented if you protect yourself from UV light. We also know that UV rays make your skin wrinkled and old-looking. How does that happen?

The cosmetic effects of sunlight and UV rays on skin (also known as photo-aging, or dermatoheliosis) manifests in three ways:

- blotchy sunspots
- loose skin
- wrinkles

Let's look at all three.

BLOTCHY SUNSPOTS

Beautiful skin is uniform in color, with pigmentation (or skin tone) even throughout. Sun-damaged skin is blotchy. UV light affects the pigment-producing cells in the skin. These cells are responsible for evenly distributing color in the skin. Over time, when exposed to excessive amounts of UV light, they literally develop "diarrhea." Instead of evenly distributing color throughout the skin, these cells spew pigment out all over the skin in uncontrolled doses, leaving the skin blotchy, spotted, and unevenly pigmented.

LOOSE SKIN

Loose, saggy skin is the result of three forces: the sun, gravity, and oxidative damage. Oxidative damage and free radicals are discussed in Commandment VI: Fight Free Radicals.

LET'S TALK ABOUT THE SUN AND GRAVITY.

As you read in the Introduction, youthful skin has good elasticity, a quality that allows it to be stretched and then easily snap back into shape. Elasticity is due to elastic-like fibers in the deeper layers of skin. Think of these as mini rubber bands below the skin.

The sun ruins the skin's rubber band–like quality by literally destroying and breaking apart these elastic-like fibers. Over time, as the skin gets pulled south by gravity, the cheeks sag, the nose sags, and the eyes sag—resulting in a droopy, bloodhound-like face.

You can't stop gravity. However, you can block the sun's rays from reaching your skin and preserve the skin's elasticity to help combat the effects of gravity on skin. The more well preserved these elastic-like fibers are, the less gravity's effect on skin and the less droopiness in the face.

WRINKLES
Try lifting your eyebrows and holding that movement so as to make your face appear surprised. You will notice the skin on your forehead wrinkles as you tense your forehead muscles.

In certain areas of the face, wrinkles on the surface of the skin are due to muscle movement below the skin. Every time muscles below the skin are flexed, the skin surface above it wrinkles up. When the muscle relaxes, the wrinkles go away. Gradually, over time, these wrinkles permanently crease the skin, and eventually wrinkles remain, even when the muscle below is not flexing. Excessive exposure to UV rays will hasten the appearance of permanent wrinkles.

Here's how:
Youthful skin—not damaged by the sun—is plump, filled with fluid made up of water, collagen (a structural protein), and normal oil gland fluid. UV light and tanning thin the skin, break down collagen, and destroy normal oil glands.

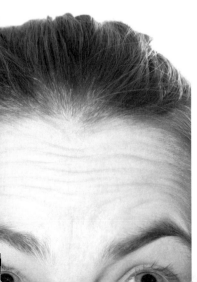

Plump, undamaged skin makes the wrinkling effect less obvious and less able to cause permanent creases in the skin surface. Thin skin makes the wrinkling effect more obvious and allows permanent creases to form on the skin's surface. (We can do something about some of those wrinkles. For details, see Commandment VII: Thou Shalt Botox, Commandment VIII: Fill 'er Up, and Commandment IX: Love Thy Laser.)

How to Choose a Sunscreen

Sunscreens come in several different forms, including lotions, creams, oils, gels, sprays, sticks, and aerosols. Whichever you choose is fine. There are two main categories of sunscreens: physical and chemical.

Physical sunscreens literally get between your skin and the sun's rays. Applying physical sunscreens is like draping an opaque, waxy coat over your skin to block light from entering. These sunscreens are usually pasty white when applied to the skin, although newer micronized versions are less pasty. The main ingredients are titanium and zinc.

Chemical sunscreens block the sun by causing complex chemical reactions that prevent light from penetrating the skin. This type of sunscreen has the advantage of blending into the skin without causing a white pasty coating, but the disadvantage is that the chemical reactions may be harmful. Chemical sunscreens should not be used in children under two.

How High Should I Go?

"My doctor told me SPF 15 was the highest I needed to go and anything more than that doesn't make a difference. Is that true?"

Well—that would be true if you lived in a lab and your skin was the subject of a sunburn experiment. But in the real world and from a practical standpoint, in my opinion such a statement is false.

Here is why: Your skin sweats and is exposed to wind, water, and contact with your hands and other objects that can physically smear or remove your sunscreen. Also, most people don't apply and reapply enough sunscreen to adequately protect their skin in the first place. (See practical sunscreen tips on page 18.)

For daily use, products with SPF 15 or 30 are adequate. On days of intense sun exposure, choose a sunscreen with the highest SPF you can tolerate. Higher SPF products are usually thicker and pastier.

WHICH TYPE OF SUNSCREEN IS BETTER?

Both are reportedly safe. I prefer physical blocking agents because they are less irritating and less likely to induce oxidative damage. However, you may choose to use either. The more important factors in your choice of sunscreen are the SPF and UV coverage.

The SPF indicates the amount of time you can spend in the sun while wearing a particular sunscreen before you get burned. For example, if a sunscreen has an SPF 15, it takes 15 times as long to get sunburned than if you had no sunscreen on at all. If a sunscreen has an SPF 30, it takes 30 times as long to get a sunburn than if you had on no sunscreen.

This is assuming, of course, that you put on enough sunscreen to cover the area you are trying to protect. (See Practical Sunscreen Tips ahead.)

"Any sunscreen is good as long as it has SPF in it, right?" Wrong.

SPF measures only one type of harmful light from the sun (UVB) and is not the only factor to consider when you choose a sunscreen. You must make sure you have adequate UVA protection as well. Let me explain.

UV light from the sun is divided into three categories—A, B, and C—based on intensity:

- UV<u>A</u>
- UV<u>B</u>
- UV<u>C</u>

The most harmful types of rays are UVA and UVB. UVC is absorbed by the ozone layer. Almost all sunscreens provide coverage to protect against UVB, and SPF is used to measure that protection only. But only a few sunscreens protect against UVA, and SPF does not account for UVA protection.

UVA is especially damaging because, unlike UVB, it can pass through glass and harm you while you are driving or sitting by a window. It is also the type of UV light that is most closely linked to melanoma, the deadly skin cancer.

The best sunscreens contain both UVA and UVB protection.

Suntan Lotion vs. Sunscreen

Don't be fooled—suntan lotion is not the same thing as sunscreen.

Most often, suntan lotions—which tend to have exotic names conjuring up tropical locations and the darkest skin imaginable—contain little or no ingredients that will protect your skin from the sun's damaging rays. Instead, suntan lotions generously invite UV rays to up your melanin output. These products are extremely dangerous because many people believe they are protected and tend to stay out in the sun even longer.

A double "no-no," these products are often used to enhance the results at a tanning salon.

FDA Calls for New Labels

In June 2011, the Food and Drug Administration issued new guidelines for sunscreen labeling to help consumers better understand the effectiveness of the products and prevent confusion.

– No sunscreen product may claim an SPF above 50.

– Sunscreens that block UVB radiation and some UVA radiation may be labeled as "broad-spectrum" products.

– Broad-spectrum products with an SPF of 15 or higher may state on the label that they reduce the risk of premature skin aging and skin cancer.

– No sunscreen may be advertised as a "sun blocker."

– Claims that products are "waterproof" or "sweat proof" must be reworded as "water resistant," and labels must state whether this protection offered lasts forty or eighty minutes.

Read the list of ingredients on the label and look for the following:

- avobenzone
- oxybenzone
- mexoryl SX
- menthyl anthranilate
- titanium dioxide
- zinc oxide

All of these ingredients cover UVA and are usually mixed with other ingredients that also cover UVB. Those last two, physical blocking sunscreens titanium dioxide and zinc oxide, cover both UVA and UVB.

Today, sunscreens indicate on the front of the package if they protect against UVA, UVB, or both. Remember: Choose a sunscreen that covers both. Sunscreens that block both types of harmful light may be labeled as broad-spectrum products.

While you are reading labels, here is something to watch out for: Products that contain "PABA" (para-aminobenzoic acid, a.k.a. Padimate O), oxybenzone (which is on the list above), or cinnamates. These ingredients are common skin allergens. Avoid them if you have sensitive skin or have allergic reactions to sunscreen.

Practical Sunscreen Tips

The obvious way to protect your skin from the sun is to apply sunscreen to areas exposed to sun, especially your face, every day, as though your life depended on it—because it may. If not your life, certainly your skin and your appearance depend on it. Patients ask me a lot of questions about sun protection.

"I put a few dabs of sunscreen on. That should do the trick, right?" Wrong.

A study conducted a few years ago revealed that most people—up to 70 percent of the population—don't apply sunscreen before going out. Those that do tend to apply only 25 to 50 percent of the recommended amount of sunscreen. Don't be one of those people.

Every day, to effectively protect the face and neck (front and back) use about one teaspoon of sunscreen. Don't forget your ears. If you are bald, grease up the dome. If your arms are exposed, coat 'em up and rub it in. Even if your arms are covered, pay extra attention to your hands.

"I'll be in the water the whole time. I don't need sunscreen, right?" Wrong.

If you are going swimming, headed to the beach, or will be in the sun all day and plan to take off your shirt, kick off your flip-flops and most of the rest of your clothing, liberally use sunscreen on your face, neck, chest, back, shoulders, arms, and legs. To adequately cover the sun-exposed areas of the body, the American Academy of Dermatology recommends that you slather on one full ounce—enough sunscreen to fill a shot glass.

This should be done thirty minutes prior to sun exposure, not when you show up at the beach or pool. Pay particular attention to the tops of your ears and feet and even in between those toes. When you get out of the water or if you've perspired a lot, dry off and reapply sunscreen. Sunburned lips sting—buy lip balm with sunscreen. Also, wear dark sunglasses to protect your eyes.

Water-Resistant Sunscreen

A great option for the avid swimmer, water-resistant sunscreens are tested to ensure SPF is still present after forty to eighty minutes of swimming. The oil base in these products makes them resistant to water but also makes them a bit greasier than other sunscreens. They should be applied thirty minutes prior to swimming. Water-resistant sunscreen should also be used during outdoor exercise or activities that will make you sweat.

"It's not even sunny out.
I won't get sunburned, right?"
Wrong.

Remember, UV rays are present on gray days as well as bright, sunny days, and we know that UV rays penetrate clouds. So if you are going outdoors on an overcast day, ignore the weather and lather up.

How to Avoid
UV Rays

On days of intense sun—especially between the hours of 10 a.m. and 3 p.m., the sun and its rays are in position to have the best shot at your skin. Still, no matter how long you are outdoors, wearing sunscreen alone may not be enough to prevent you from getting sunburned.

It's always best to outsmart the sun and adopt "sun-avoidance" techniques. This doesn't mean you have to become a vampire and stay in until dark or never go to the beach or hide in your home. Sun-avoidance techniques allow you to have a healthy outdoor life while at the same time preventing sunburn and photo-aging.

Here are some tips:
- Wear a hat with a brim that shades your face.
- When possible, sit under an umbrella or in the shade.
- Avoid aiming your face directly at the sun.

You already know that a tank top or cut-off T-shirt won't offer your body much protection while you play beach volleyball. On the other hand, who wants to wear a long-sleeved, dark blue flannel to the beach? Choose lightweight clothing that covers most of your body.

Another option is sun-protective clothing, which is clothing made from fabric treated to reduce exposure to UVB and UVA rays. Typically, this clothing is made from fabrics made with a dense, tight weave and comes in colors that help block additional rays.

Sun-protective clothing carries an Ultraviolet Protection Factor (UPF), usually from a UPF 15 to UPF 50+. UPF is a measurement typically used for fabrics, unlike SPF, which is a measurement for topically applied products. UPF measures the amount of UV rays that pass through the fabric and get to the skin. In other words, a shirt made from fabric with a rating of 50 will allow only 1/50th of the sun's UV rays to reach your skin.

The Skin Cancer Foundation awards its Seal of Recommendation to some sun-protective clothing that offers a minimum UPF 30. The agency ranks a UPF rating of 30–49 as "very good protection" and 50+ as "excellent protection." If you have a favorite sun-protective shirt or pair of shorts, remember that frequent washing will lessen the effectiveness of the treated fabric.

Speaking of washing, there are facial cleansers on the market that claim to provide some SPF coverage when you wash your face. Another option is makeup or foundation that contain SPF. These are good options for day-to-day use, but I wouldn't count on them for protection during intense, prolonged sun exposure.

Commercial laundry additives are also available that contain sunscreen. When you add it to your laundry, the additive is said to wash a UPF 30 into the garments. The additive is advertised to last in the clothing through twenty washings.

Skiers Beware

Sunburns don't happen just at the beach, on the water, or on the tennis court. Because of the higher altitude and light reflected off snow, skiers are also susceptible. Use common sense—and sunscreen—on the slopes. Here are some guidelines:

– Wear high-SPF broad-spectrum sunscreen on your face and hands.

– Wear high-SPF broad-spectrum sunscreen on your ears if they are exposed.

– Wear lip balm with sunscreen on your lips.

– Wear dark sunglasses to protect your eyes.

Sunlight
and Vitamin D

Some people (and unfortunately some of them are doctors) think, "Lying out is good for me so that I get my vitamin D."

These people justify baking in the sun to capture the benefits of vitamin D and completely ignore the risk of deadly skin cancers caused by UV light, not to mention the cosmetic effects of photo-aging. The controversial recommendation to bask in the sun was sparked after several studies linked vitamin D levels to internal cancer and disease prevention, although the National Institutes of Health did not show a correlation between the level of vitamin D and overall cancer mortality for most types of cancer.

The tanning bed industry's multimillion-dollar marketing efforts to falsely state the facts about vitamin D and sunlight furthered this debate in the wrong direction. Several other companies, including some doctors promoting "doctor-recommended" products, joined the paper chase, selling sunlamps for home use that are intended to boost your body's vitamin D with artificial UV light—the same harmful rays found in tanning beds and natural sunlight.

Here's the truth:
Vitamin D is naturally produced in the skin, and UV light is necessary for this process, but the amount of time your skin needs to make vitamin D is very short—say five to ten minutes a day, three days a week. You will get sufficient vitamin D when sunlight shines on your skin for that brief period of time.

It is better to limit this short amount of unprotected sun exposure to the arms, legs, chest, or back. To avoid the effects of photo-aging, leave your face out of it—maybe smiling from under a broad-brimmed hat.

Or, to avoid the harmful effects of unprotected sunlight altogether, you can obtain adequate vitamin D through foods such as milk, oily fish (salmon, tuna, herring, catfish), mushrooms, egg yolks, and in supplement form. For most people I recommend a daily supplement of 1000 IU of vitamin D3. (New studies suggest higher doses of vitamin D may be beneficial, but the jury is still out.) For a complete list of supplement recommendations, see Skin Commandment VI: Fight Free Radicals.

Although rare, vitamin D deficiency is more likely to occur in dark-skinned individuals, elderly persons, people with medical conditions that limit their sun exposure, obese individuals, or those with fat absorption problems. These individuals should consult with their doctors about vitamin D supplements and continue to use sunscreen and sun-avoidance techniques. Research continues to determine the best levels of vitamin D and the beneficial effects, if any, or the detrimental effects of high doses.

Even Tone

Here are some tips for using self-tanners to ensure a natural, uniformly bronze color throughout:

- Always cleanse and gently exfoliate your skin before application.
- If you plan to shave, do it beforehand.
- Use an applicator or cotton ball to avoid dyeing the palms of your hands.
- Use less product on the face and more product on the body.
- Use a blow dryer (set on cool) immediately after application to dry the product.
- Use tinted sunscreen to help maintain your bronze glow while providing protection from UV rays.

Bronzers, Sunless Tanning Lotions, and Spray Tans: A Safer Bet

"I love how my skin looks when it is tan or has some color. Can I use a bronzer, sunless tanning lotion, or get a spray tan?"

Yes. These methods temporarily "dye" the outer skin layer without exposing the skin to harmful UV rays from the sun or tanning beds. They have no reported harmful effects and may be used in conjunction with any anti-aging or skin enhancement program, except before certain laser treatments. Check with your dermatologist.

Use them as much as you like, but remember: NO TANNING.

Tanning pills and injections that are designed to increase your body's own melanin production are also available. However, they are potentially dangerous, not well studied, and not approved by the FDA.

23

The Unbreakable Skin Commandment

Thou Shalt Not Tan is the most important skin health and beauty rule, and one that must be followed. I hope that before reading another word of this book, every individual genuinely interested in enhancing or maintaining healthy skin makes a commitment to the first Skin Commandment. Without adhering to this most basic of skin-care rules, you will find that the other nine Skin Commandments are a waste of your time.

Without the sun—an orb that civilizations have worshipped for thousands of years—this planet could not sustain life. Worship if you must, but wear sunscreen and protect yourself appropriately, especially your "money maker"—your face. I'm not saying the sun can't be your friend—just not your BFF all day, every day.

SKIN II COMMANDMENT

HONOR THY SKIN

OBEYING SKIN COMMANDMENT II

Build your skin-care regimen around the basics:
Wear sunscreen, cleanse, hydrate, and exfoliate your skin.

Do not pop pimples, pick your skin,
or poke your face with needles.

Touch your face as little as possible.

Avoid home remedies and skin-care gadgets
that may irritate your skin.

Avoid skin-care products with fragrances,
bright colors, and allergenic preservatives.

Be gentle with your skin.

Your skin is a precious possession, one worth caring for, in the hope that it will guard you, protect you, and maintain your health and beauty throughout your life. Yet sometimes, people go overboard when it comes to skin care, especially on the face. Others pick on themselves, both literally and figuratively.

The second Skin Commandment is a direct order to stop!

The best way to Honor Thy Skin is to keep it simple and take a "hands-off" approach more often than not. Let's get specific.

BASIC SKIN CARE
Basic skin care can be summed up briefly: _____

- wear sunscreen
- cleanse
- moisturize
- exfoliate

These four elements are so important they have their own dedicated chapters in this book. Here are quick summaries.

Skin Commandment I: Thou Shalt Not Tan states clearly the first line of defense when caring for your skin. Wear sunscreen on sun-exposed areas when you go out in the sun. Wear sunscreen when you go out on cloudy days, too. Wear sunscreen on your face and neck. Always. Period.

Next, cleanliness matters. I'll cover that in depth in Skin Commandment III: Cleanse Correctly. I recommend you cleanse your face two times a day, plus an extra time or two if you have oily skin or if you have perspired a great deal—maybe at the gym, doing yoga, or kickboxing.

Next, proper hydration is important. That's covered thoroughly in Skin Commandment IV: Hydrate Holistically, where I'll make recommendations to help you moisturize your skin and hydrate your body efficiently and effectively.

Fourth, exfoliation helps speed up cell renewal and leaves your skin looking younger, fresher, and more radiant. It may also reverse sun damage and prevent certain forms of skin cancer. For details on exfoliating at home or at your dermatologist's office, see Skin Commandment V: Exfoliate Effectively.

Now that we know the basics, let's look at other ways to Honor Thy Skin.

POPPING, PICKING, AND PROBING

First things first. Please—never pick at your face with your nails, needles, or any other sharp object. This behavior is not only neurotic, but also extremely destructive to your skin. Many people with permanent acne scars have caused the scars themselves by picking. Don't do it.

Turn to a professional. Board-certified dermatologists and licensed aestheticians, using specialized, sterile instruments, can remove blackheads and skin debris for you. Think about it. You wouldn't trust yourself to remove your own gallbladder, so don't perform minor surgery on your skin.

Who among us hasn't stood in front of a mirror and pondered popping, picking, or probing a problematic pimple?

The key to understanding why you shouldn't resort to any of those actions is to first understand pimples. A pimple is a collection of fluid beneath the skin surface caused by overactive oil glands. Certain bacteria that thrive and feed on this excess oil

**Dr. T's Tips:
Save Your Neck**

Here's an important skin-care tip: Whatever you do to care for your face— apply sun block, cleanse, or hydrate— do the same for your neck and chest, too. It's easy to overlook those areas. If you don't want your décolletage to age more quickly than your face, put "care for your neck and chest" on your to-do list now.

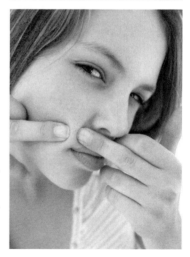

begin to grow. The growth of bacteria causes white blood cells (the kind that fight bacteria) from your immune system to also enter the oil gland. That is the whitehead or white "pus" in the pimple.

Think of a balloon of bacteria, oil, and white pus under your skin. If the balloon is squeezed, it will burst, spilling out fluid. If there is no tunnel to the outside of the skin and it doesn't flow out easily, the balloon will literally implode, or explode inwardly. When a pimple implodes, bacteria, pus, and oil all form in new places under your skin, which allows more white blood cells to enter your skin. Then you are left with even more pus under the skin, which can lead to a big infection. Unfortunately, these skin infections can lead to permanent scarring.

Still think it's a good idea to mess with pimples?

If you are not convinced, and you are determined to proceed—if you MUST pop—then please follow these guidelines:

Wait until the pimple is white on its surface (whitehead), so you know if you pop it, fluid will easily flow outward and not implode on the inside, spreading bacteria and pus. These types of pimples may be gently pressed to extrude pus.

If a pimple is red and inflamed (not showing white pus on the surface), I advise you to leave it alone. Don't touch it or squeeze it. Your dermatologist can get rid of the pimple for you with an injection. Or if you must take action, apply a warm compress to allow the fluid within that pimple to "come to a head." To make a warm compress, immerse a small hand towel in hot water and wring it out. The towel should be warm—not piping hot—tolerable to the skin without burning.

Once a whitehead is visible at the skin's surface (which may take several days), you may gently apply pressure and extrude the fluid.

Banishing Zits Forever

Maybe you are starting to agree with me about the importance of leaving pimples alone, but maybe you wonder how to avoid getting pimples in the first place. No single practice is guaranteed to leave you pimple free, especially if you have oily skin, but there are simple ways to help protect your skin from breakouts.

Cleanliness matters! CLEAN skin is more likely to be CLEAR skin. I'm not talking about just washing your face. You can carefully wash your face and then undo your efforts without realizing it. Many people have the terrible habit of resting their faces on their hands while sitting. You've seen this often, in classrooms or boardroom settings, whenever someone is seated for an extended period of time.

Maybe you've even been guilty of "sitting on your face" yourself. The next time you start to put your chin in your hand, think about how many doorknobs, stair railings, faucets, dollar bills, and other dirty, bacteria-ridden objects your hands have touched throughout the day. Did you shake hands with anyone? That counts too. So does leaning your chin on a phone that likely carries residue from makeup or bacteria from dirty hands.

Imagine subjecting your facial skin to direct contact with that dirt and bacteria for an hour or more while sitting at your desk at work or in a classroom. When you touch your face, you are literally implanting microbes and filth into your pores, creating a petri dish for bacteria to grow on your face.

As a general rule, after cleansing and applying products, try not to touch your face at all, and definitely don't "sit on your face."

At one time, teenagers were told that pizza was the primary cause of pimples. That turned out not to be the whole story, though certain foods do affect your skin. Because your skin reflects your general health, eating right, exercising, sleeping well, and reducing stress all can help keep your skin healthy and your face clear. More about all of that in Skin Commandment VI: Fight Free Radicals, and Skin Commandment X: Live Healthy.

Other Perpetrators of Pimples

– hair in your face

– headbands, tight-fitting hats, and other constricting headgear

– old makeup, heavily applied makeup, and dirty makeup applicators

– oil-based cosmetics, moisturizers, and sunscreens

Home Remedies

Patients constantly ask me about "sure-fire" home remedies.
For instance: ─────────────────────────────

"Should I put toothpaste on my pimples?" **No.**

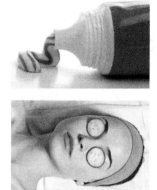

"I saw this battery-powered thing in a magazine that "zaps" zits using an electric current. Does it work?" **No.**

"My mom told me to rub mayonnaise on my face to prevent wrinkles. Does that work?" **No.**

"Does milk lighten my skin tone and help get rid of dark spots?" **No.**

Should I use bacitracin or Neosporin® on a rash or for dry skin? **No.**

"If I place two cucumber slices over my eyes while I sleep, will I get rid of dark circles?" **No.**

"Can I use lemon juice and sunlight to bleach my skin"? **No.**

No, no, no, no, and yet again, no.

Don't Act Rashly

Two of the most common over-the-counter products used to treat rashes or for skin lubrication are bacitracin and Neosporin®. Bacitracin and neomycin (one of the active ingredients in Neosporin®) are two of the most allergenic ingredients on the market and can cause severe skin reactions.

Next time you reach for one of these products, think twice—you may be doing more harm than good. If you have a rash, consult your dermatologist. For proper ways to hydrate your skin, see Skin Commandment IV: Hydrate Holistically.

I've heard them all, an unending list of unbelievable home remedies that many of my patients use regularly—all to no avail. My answer to all of them is simple: Don't do it. None of these treatments do anything to help your skin.

Some of them may seem to work at first. Toothpaste will dry out your pimples, but it will break the skin's surface and will potentially cause infection and scarring. And some are just bad from the get-go. Lemon juice when exposed to your skin in combination with sunlight causes a severe blistering rash. These home remedies all are unsafe, old-school treatments that are simply bad for your skin.

AVOID IRRITATING PRODUCTS

When it comes to skin-care products, less is best. In general, they should be bland. Products with additives that can cause irritation are a definite DON'T. Many people who have chronically itchy skin, inflamed red skin, or chronic hives may be having an allergic skin reaction to an additive in one of their skin-care products.

Here's a bad idea I hear frequently:

"I'm going to buy a new moisturizer that smells like cucumber, watermelon, cinnamon, or raspberries."

While they might smell good, products with strong fragrances are not good for your skin. Scented products contain chemicals that can dry out and irritate your skin.

More than 5,000 fragrances are in use today in cosmetics and skin-care products, and those fragrances are the fourth most common among all allergens, according to the North American Contact Dermatitis Group. Fragrances account for 11.7 percent of all allergic skin rashes known as contact dermatitis. Another organization, the American Contact Dermatitis Society, named fragrance the Allergen of the Year in 2007.

Odiferous Allergens

Here is a list of fragrance additives to watch out for, especially if you have allergic or sensitive skin:

- balsam of Peru
  (a.k.a. myroxylon pereirae)
- oak moss
- cinnamic aldehyde
- cinnamic alcohol
- alpha amyl cinnamic alcohol
- geraniol
- hydroxycitronellal
- isoeugenol
- eugenol

- colophony
- benzyl acetate
- benzyl alcohol
- lyral
- citral
- farnesol
- coumarin
- citronellol
- alpha-hexyl cinnamal

Don't think that choosing a product advertised as "unscented" will solve the problem. Unscented products often contain a fragrance developed to mask the others. Look for products labeled "fragrance-free" to avoid allergic skin reactions.

Here's another common misconception. "This cream is really good for my skin because it comes from a natural plant."

The term "natural"—very popular these days—can be misleading. "Natural" is used in advertising to imply that a product is somehow superior to other products, but that is not always the case. Although many natural ingredients are beneficial, some are harmful.

Think about ordinary plants that are toxic to the skin, such as poison ivy. Just because something is produced naturally doesn't mean it's good. More important than whether something is natural is if the ingredients have been scientifically proven to help your skin. Many beneficial natural products with excellent scientific data are available, and I am all for them. More about those later. (See Skin Commandment IV: Hydrate Holistically and Skin Commandment VI: Fight Free Radicals.)

Color is great for fashion, but if your skin-care products are electric blue, purple, red, orange, or any other bright color, get rid of them. They likely contain large amounts of artificial dyes that also can be harmful to your skin.

Dyes are used in cosmetics to produce an appearance appealing to customers and also to neutralize any undesirable colors from the combination of ingredients. People with sensitive skin are particularly susceptible to irritation from these dyes, but they may cause a reaction in others as well. Always choose white, cream, and pale, lightly tinted cosmetic products that are more likely to contain only trace amounts of coloring agent.

Maybe you brought home a fragrance-free product with no perceptible dyes. Is it okay for you to use?

Maybe. Maybe not.

The product may be loaded with allergenic preservatives. Preservatives are used in cosmetic products to kill microorganisms (like fungus and bacteria), inhibit their growth, and prevent skin infections. The American Academy of Dermatology names preservatives in cosmetics and skin-care products as the second most common cause of skin allergies. Unfortunately, it is almost impossible to get around preservatives because products that contain no preservatives have an extremely short shelf life. They simply don't last.

The Food and Drug Administration has ruled that many preservatives are deemed safe in small amounts. However, certain types of allergy-causing preservatives should be on your radar if you have sensitive or allergy-prone skin.

Problematic Preservatives

Here are some preservative ingredients that I suggest you keep an eye out for, especially if you have sensitive or allergic skin:

- quaternium 15
- dimethyl-dimethyl
  (DMDM) hydantoin
- imidazolidinyl urea
- diazolidinyl urea
- 2-bromo-2-nitropropane-1, 3-diol
- kathon CG
- thimerasol
- para-phenylenediamine

The first five belong to a class of preservatives called formaldehyde releasers and are among the most common causes of allergic skin reactions. Thimerasol contains mercury, a toxic element. Para-phenylenediamine can be found in hair dyes and also is a common skin allergy-causing culprit. All of these preservatives may cause allergic reactions, inflammation, and damage to your skin.

Cancer-Causing Ingredients in Cosmetics?

Preservatives called parabens have been the subject of much controversy when a study published in the *Journal of Applied Toxicology* in 2004 detected trace amounts of parabens in breast tumors.

Studies also revealed that parabens weakly mimic estrogen, which is the major hormone in many breast cancers. However, many other common ingredients mimic estrogen as well, including phytoestrogens, for example, which are found in soy products. Additional studies found no conclusive proof that topically applied parabens cause breast cancer.

Another common ingredient that stirred a cancer frenzy is Sodium Laurel Sulfate (SLS), a detergent used at low concentrations in shampoos. To date, no substantial evidence has linked SLS or any of the chemicals in the same category (referred to as "sulfates") to cancer.

The fear of parabens and sulfates has certainly been overhyped and sensationalized by the media. It should be noted, however, that the long-term effects of parabens and sulfates are unknown. Many people prefer to avoid them whenever possible, although parabens are found in many food preservatives and sulfates are found in other personal hygiene products like toothpaste and soap.

The bottom line about skin-care products: A good skin-care product has no aroma, no bright colors, no irritating preservatives, and is gentle on your skin. Avoiding these additives prevents unnecessary free radical damage to your skin cells, which keeps them healthy and beautiful. I'll explain this in more detail in Skin Commandment VI: Fight Free Radicals, where I offer suggestions on how to decrease your overall oxidative stress load.

Exfoliating Tools:
The Good, the Bad, and the Ugly

A plethora of skin-care products are available to help you exfoliate dead skin from every part of your body. Often, these products are misused and the skin ends up irritated and abused, especially on the face.

WHAT'S OUT THERE?
Let's start with cleansers loaded with mini-crystals or so-called "buffing grains," which are used commonly to treat acne or remove dead skin. Some people figure if a little is good, more is better. They apply large amounts of the "buffing" product to their faces and scrub vigorously, as though they were cleaning out the tub or sink.

These products can scratch your skin like a diamond on glass and should be avoided entirely.

Devices that are used to polish your face, like battery-powered electric face brushes sold on infomercials, are no better.

These products, in theory, may make sense, but the bristles used on most of these instruments are far too harsh for the skin on your face and should be avoided. Stay tuned for gentler, non-abrasive facial brushes. In the meantime, Honor Thy Skin.

Skin-Care Gifts from the Earth

A form of volcanic rock born in the intense heat of a volcano, pumice stones have now found their way into our homes as part of our skin-care regimens.

Used for centuries by the ancient Egyptians, loofahs are made from dried tropical vines. They are sold as back brushes, mitts, and small scrubbers for exfoliating the skin.

Natural sponges are made from multi-cellular sea creatures that look like plants, but most body sponges available are made from cellulose foam or polyurethane foam.

Certain parts of the body, other than the face, can handle a good scrubbing, but don't overdo it. The key is to be gentle and always use finesse. Used with a soft circular motion on damp skin, pumice stones may be used on your heels and the soles (not the tops) of your feet to remove dead or callused skin. Loofahs, soft-bristled brushes, soft sponges, and shower scrunchies—gently used on your arms, legs, back, or chest—will help keep your skin smooth and beautiful. More to come about these and other exfoliation methods in Skin Commandment V: Exfoliate Effectively.

Again, none of these products—under any circumstances—may be used on your face. When you cleanse your face, reach for a soft washcloth. For more information on how to properly cleanse the face, see Skin Commandment III: Cleanse Correctly.

More sophisticated methods, more controlled ways of exfoliating dead skin from the face, are available at your dermatologist's office, including:

- prescription creams
- chemical peels
- dermabrasion
- laser resurfacing

For more information about these methods, see Skin Commandment V: Exfoliate Effectively and Skin Commandment IX: Love Thy Laser.

Meanwhile, Honor Thy Skin.

A Salute to Skin

Overdoing it with skin care is always a bad idea. Simplicity is key. The average person's skin weighs between six and nine pounds, and these particular pounds have an especially important job to do. So always Honor Thy Skin, and be as gentle as possible with your body's largest, most beautiful organ.

SKIN III COMMANDMENT

CLEANSE CORRECTLY

OBEYING SKIN COMMANDMENT III

For all skin types, choose a gentle cleanser without strong fragrances, bright colored dyes, allergenic preservatives, or harmful mini-crystals.

Choose a gentle cleanser for normal skin, a moisturizing cleanser for dry skin, and an exfoliating or medicated cleanser for oily or acne-prone skin.

Use a smooth-textured washcloth or clean hands.

Wash gently with warm water—never hot—and avoid long showers or baths.

Cleanse your face twice a day, in the morning and at night.

Cleanse your face more often if you have oily skin or after participating in activities that increase dirt and oil.

Cleanse less often if you have dry skin, and use a damp washcloth to remove dirt and oil instead.

Always remove makeup and rinse out hair products before bed.

Let's face it—clean, healthy, well-maintained skin exudes beauty and confidence. Add a big smile and you're going to attract all the right kinds of attention, personally and professionally.

So do you really need to read a whole chapter to know that you should wash your face? Maybe not—but here you also will learn exactly why and how to cleanse your skin.

Your skin produces its own natural moisturizer comprising proteins, lipids, and a natural moisturizing factor. These important molecules keep your outer surface cells healthy, moist, and supple so your skin does not become dry and flaky. They also prevent water from evaporating through the skin surface.

During adolescence, the oil glands go into overdrive due to raging hormones, producing excessive amounts of oil, which can lead to acne. By the time you turn twenty, oil production usually begins to slow down. With each decade to follow, the oil glands and other natural moisturizing mechanisms become less effective, leaving you with more of the responsibility for moisturizing. (For tips on moisturizing at any age, see Skin Commandment IV: Hydrate Holistically.)

Determining when and how to cleanse your skin is something of a balancing act. Everything depends on how much natural moisturizer your skin produces. Do you have normal skin? Do you have oily skin? Do you have dry skin? The answers to these questions determine the right cleansing regimen for you.

I see patients all the time with variations on these three skin types. To complicate matters more, some people have a combination of both oily and dry skin—oily in some places and dry in others. "One size fits all" simply does not apply, because you also need to factor in your age, daily activities, and occupation.

Let's begin with this simple tip: For normal skin, I recommend cleansing your face two times a day, every day—once in the morning and once before you go to bed.

Washing your face removes excess oil, dirt, and other pollutants that have collected there. Some days—days when more filthy build up occurs—you may need to add a third cleansing. For instance, you will want to wash your face more often under these circumstances: _____

- after rigorous physical activity or exercise
- after being exposed to grime on the job depending on your occupation (e.g., painter, factory worker, lab worker, etc.)
- after touring a smoggy city
- after exposure to sea air at the beach or on a boat
- after swimming laps in a chlorinated pool or salt water
- after being on an airplane
- after sitting in an air conditioned room for a long period of time

Regardless of your daily activity, oily skin must be cleansed more frequently. Excess oil builds up all day and should be removed with a third (and sometimes even a fourth) cleanse, depending on the extent of the oiliness. This may be achieved with regular cleansing or with oil-removing pads.

Older skin and dry skin should be cleansed less often, because older skin and dry skin produce less natural moisturizer and are prone to irritation and cracking. To avoid over-drying the skin, use a damp washcloth to remove dirt in the morning and at night.

No Rough Stuff

Some people think the way to make sure their face is really clean is to scrub until it's bright red.

These folks are mistaken.

In Skin Commandment II: Honor Thy Skin, I talk about the importance of being gentle with your skin. The skin on your face is extremely delicate and sensitive. If you scrub your face with anything rough, you may end up with irritation and redness.

You don't need a high-powered electric face brush or a cleanser with mini-crystals. Use a soft, open-weave (smooth-textured) clean washcloth for the face.

For the body, a soft-bristle brush, shower scrunchie, sponge, or loofah may be used gently. Or you may choose to use just your hands.

This should go without saying, but I won't risk it. If you wash your face with your hands, be sure to wash your hands before you begin in order to remove any dirt or bacteria that may have collected there. After all, there is no point in transferring dirt from your hands to your face while in the process of cleansing.

This should also go without saying, but I'm obviously not a risk taker. Hand cleansers and hand sanitizers should never be used on the face. These products contain alcohol and other harsh antiseptic ingredients that are intended to disinfect the thick skin on your hands, not your face. Because the hands are exposed to germs all day, they require a more aggressive disinfectant than other areas of your skin, especially the face.

If you decide to use a washcloth or other washing tool, be sure to also wash or replace it frequently so it does not become a reservoir for bacteria.

Too Wet Can Equal Too Dry

Some people cleanse under this false assumption: "The longer I stay in the shower, and the hotter the water temperature, the cleaner and better it is for my skin."

They are wrong.

Though it is counterintuitive, water, especially hot water, dehydrates skin. Think about how wrinkled and "prune-like" your fingers look after a long bath or after soaking in a hot tub.

Water also will strip your skin of the natural moisturizers your skin produces. So don't spend a lot of time in water— and easy does it on water temperature. Always wash your skin with warm or tepid water—never hot.

Choosing a Cleanser

Before choosing the right cleanser for your skin type, you need to understand what goes into a cleansing product. Cleansers—including the stuff you use to cleanse your face, wash your dishes, or de-grime the bathtub—all contain a main ingredient called a surfactant (a word that combines "surface" and "active") that removes surface dirt and oil. Whether the grime is on your skin, toilet, or frying pan, the surfactant literally gets the ball (or in this case the dirt and oil) rolling. The surfactant is usually a harsh chemical, one made to combat grease, oil, and dirt.

Obviously, using a strong surfactant on your stainless steel sink makes sense. Using the same ingredient on your face does not. In skin care, the better or stronger the surfactant, the more harmful to your skin, because your skin has natural moisturizers that you don't want to completely remove. Other ingredients in cleansers may include perfumes, which add aroma, and humectants, which add a moisturizing quality. Some cleansers also include ingredients that combat acne or exfoliate dead skin.

In the previous chapter, I recommended that you avoid skin-care products that contain strong fragrances and bright colored dyes, and that you be aware of allergy-causing preservatives. Cleansing products with these additives all have the potential to irritate skin.

SAY "NO" TO SOAP

See that forest green, pine-scented bar of soap in your shower stall? Throw it in the trash immediately. Under no circumstances do you want to use that on your face—or the rest of your body, for that matter.

Soap is far too harsh and drying for the skin. Though we use the word (incorrectly) to refer to all types of cleansers, the term "soap" is very specific. Not all cleansers are soaps, as you will read in a minute.

So what's wrong with soap?

The process of making soap, called saponification, involves an alkaline substance combined with oil. The final product, alkyl carboxylate, is very good at removing dirt and oil but extremely harmful to the skin's surface, stripping it of important proteins, fats, and other natural moisturizing agents. Also, because soap leaves a thick residue, it throws off the skin's normal pH, making it too alkaline, and resulting in irritated, dry—often cracked—skin.

That said, not all cleansing bars are soap. Some "non-soap" cleansing bars, like the ones shown on the cover of this book, are made with processes that do not involve saponification. Others may be made with additives such as glycerol, a moisturizing agent that combats the over-drying effects of soap.

Syndet bars (synthetic detergent bars), for example, are made with ingredients formulated in the neutral pH range. These cleansing bars are gentle and I much prefer them to soap.

Liquid non-soap cleansers (those that do not contain alkyl carboxylate) also are far less irritating and gentler on the skin than soap. The ingredients in these cleansers are usually formulated in the neutral pH range. One advantage of liquid over bar cleansers, is that more ingredients—moisturizers, exfoliators, and acne medications—can easily be mixed in.

Dr. T's Tip

Ditch your cleanser if it contains these ingredients commonly found in regular soap bars: sodium tallowate, sodium cocoate, sodium palmate.

LET YOUR SKIN TYPE LEAD THE WAY

Choose a cleanser based on your skin type. And remember—a good cleanser can smell nice, but should not be overwhelmingly fragrant.

For normal skin, consider using a lightweight syndet bar or liquid cleanser advertised as "gentle" or "mild" that simply removes dirt and oil without irritating your skin. Syndet bars contain ingredients such as:

- sodium cocoyl isethionate
- sodium cocoyl monoglyceride sulfate
- alkyl glyceryl ether sulfonate

For dry skin, consider using a thick, creamy, moisturizing liquid cleanser that removes dirt and oil and also soothes your skin. Moisturizing ingredients include glycerin, petrolatum, and dimethicone. These and other moisturizing ingredients will be discussed in the next chapter, Skin Commandment IV: Hydrate Holistically.

For oily skin or acne-prone skin, consider using a cleanser with active ingredients such as salicylic acid, glycolic acid, or a combination of both. These ingredients exfoliate dead skin, remove excess oil, and unclog pores.

Consider modest use of these types of exfoliating cleansers, too, if your goal is to combat fine lines and pigmentation due to aging and sun damage. These and other exfoliating methods will be discussed in detail in Skin Commandment V: Exfoliate Effectively. Acne-prone skin also benefits from cleansers with benzoyl peroxide, an antibiotic ingredient that kills the bacteria that causes acne. Caution: Overuse of benzoyl peroxide can lead to oxidative damage and premature aging of the skin, so only use it if you have active acne. Avoid it if you do not. See Skin Commandment VI: Fight Free Radicals.

"I bought a facial cleanser that promises to clear my acne. Will it? **Probably not.**

If you buy a cleanser that promises to completely clear acne, obliterate wrinkles or get rid of sunspots, these promises are likely empty ones.

Washing your face with any kind of cleanser is considered "short-contact therapy," something that you apply and then immediately wash off. The effects of cleansers on acne or wrinkles can be helpful, but are modest at best. Again, the goal of cleansing your skin is to remove dirt and excess oil, and "miracle" cleansing products that profess to do anything dramatic really cannot make good on the promise.

If you are concerned about acne, see your dermatologist. If worrying about wrinkles keeps you up at night, see Skin Commandment VII: Thou Shalt Botox. If sunspots are your greatest nemesis, see Skin Commandment V: Exfoliate Effectively and Skin Commandment IX: Love Thy Laser.

In Skin Commandment VI: Fight Free Radicals, I explain the benefits of using skin-care products that contain antioxidants, which can prevent damage to your skin and protect you from some signs of aging. The details are all on the pages ahead, but here is a quick-hit list of topical antioxidants that have been proven to help protect your skin.

If you wish to include antioxidants in your cleanser as part of your skin-care regimen, I recommend that you look for a cleansing product that contains one or more of the following:

- vitamin A
- vitamin C
- vitamin E
- CO-enzyme Q10 (CO-Q10)
- green tea

Going for the Combo

If you have combination skin—oily in some areas and dry in others—use different cleansing products for different parts of your face and body. In general, your facial skin, especially the "T-zone" area (forehead and nose), is usually oilier than most parts of your body.

No matter which cleanser you choose, pay attention to its effects on your face. If your face feels excessively tight (a little tightness is normal) and dry or appears red and irritated after washing, your skin is alerting you to choose a gentler product. After cleansing, your face should feel clean, smooth, and soft.

In the morning, wash your face before applying sunscreen or makeup. At night, before you wash your face, you'll want to remove your makeup. In keeping with my theme of being gentle with your skin, I urge you to choose nonabrasive makeup-removal products.

Look for makeup remover advertised as "mild" or "gentle." Whether you buy a cream, liquid, or makeup "wipes," remove your makeup gently and carefully, especially around your eyes. To remove eye makeup, dampen a cotton ball with a mild eye makeup remover. Slowly stroke it over your eyelid. The skin on your eyelids is even thinner than that on your face, so this is no place for harsh rubbing. If you wear a lot of mascara or eye shadow, you may need to use a second fresh cotton ball or a damp cotton swab.

Now you are ready to Cleanse Correctly.

A small dab—about a half-teaspoon—of liquid cleanser or a handful of suds from a syndet bar cleanser mixed with water should do it. Apply the cleanser to your face in a gentle, circular motion using a smooth-textured washcloth or your clean hands. Continue gently spreading the suds evenly on the face for about thirty seconds, taking time to remove dirt and oil and allowing the active ingredients to penetrate and do their job. Rinse with warm water until all of the suds are completely removed, leaving no residue on the skin. Gently pat your face dry with a clean, soft towel—no enthusiastic scrubbing is required.

Dr. T's Warm-to-Cool Cleansing Tip

Here's a simple cleansing tip to firm up and soothe your facial skin. After cleansing correctly with cleanser and warm water, turn the water temperature to cold for a quick, final rinse. Cold water causes your blood vessels to tighten, calms inflammation, and leaves the face feeling firm and fresh.

"But isn't scrubbing my face the only way to open my pores and clean them out?"

No. Unlike doors, pores don't open or close, and the size of your pores is mostly determined by genetics. Aggressive scrubbing only serves to irritate your face.

The Next Steps

What happens next? That depends on the type of skin you have.

If you have acne, oily skin, or clogged pores, you may want to follow cleansing with a toner. Certain toners remove any additional oily residue and also can act as an exfoliater. For instance, a salicylic toner helps exfoliate dead skin, dislodge blackheads, and remove excess oil. (For more detailed information on exfoliation products and treatments, see Skin Commandment V: Exfoliate Effectively.)

Again, you want to apply the toner with gentle strokes. You are not waxing furniture here, and your goal is not to remove every bit of the natural moisturizing factor, oils, or proteins from your skin. Those important molecules work to protect your skin, and you don't want to put them out of a job.

The next step is to hydrate your skin. Skin Commandment IV: Hydrate Holistically provides detailed information about how to best do this.

Another Important Step

Hair products—such as gel, mousse, and hairspray—all can clog your pores and lead to breakouts when these products migrate from your hair to your pillowcase to your face as you sleep.

The best way to avoid this contact with harmful chemicals is to rinse any products out of your hair before you go to bed.

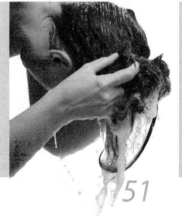

51

Closing
Cleansing Comments

Correctly cleansing your face every day is a good investment in your skin health and beauty. Make a commitment to that investment, and promise yourself that you will never skip this important step. If you stick to your promise, you—and everyone else—will see the payoff.

SKIN
COMMANDMENT
IV

HYDRATE HOLISTICALLY

OBEYING SKIN COMMANDMENT IV

For all skin types, choose a moisturizer without strong fragrances, brightly colored dyes, or allergenic preservatives.

For normal skin, moisturize with a water-based product twice a day, in the morning and at night.

For oily skin or acne-prone skin, moisturize once a day—in the morning—with an oil-free product that contains sunscreen.

For dry skin, moisturize with an oil-based product on the body and a water-based product on the face frequently throughout the day.

Apply moisturizer while your skin is damp.

Hydrate from within by drinking plenty of water and increasing your consumption of raw, water-rich, plant-based foods.

Avoid excess alcohol and caffeine consumption.

In medical school, the first time you examine someone, you are taught to tug on the skin of a patient's hand or arm and then watch how quickly the skin retracts when you let go. This quick test determines skin turgor.

Skin turgor is a direct measurement of internal hydration. Skin that snaps back indicates a healthy, well-hydrated body. Skin that stays "tented" and retracts slowly indicates dehydration. You may have seen your veterinarian perform this quick test on your pet. In extreme cases, poor skin turgor may indicate a medical emergency. Most often, hydrating your skin from within is no emergency, but it makes good sense to do so.

Some doctors—even some dermatologists—may tell you that staying hydrated does not affect your skin. That's simply not true. Many people also have the misconception that dry skin is an indication of internal dehydration. That's not true either.

Water provides many important services for the human body. Keeping up your fluid intake will help keep your body functioning smoothly and keep your skin healthy and beautiful. Some foods also hydrate the body and may help reverse signs of aging. Details will come later in this chapter. For now, grab a tall glass of water, and let's talk about hydrating from without, using topical moisturizing creams.

Rubbing It In

The outermost layer of the skin—the stratum corneum—works as a barrier to keep out foreign substances. This also is the layer that appears cracked and flaky when skin is dry, or silky smooth when skin is well hydrated.

The natural moisturizing mechanism built into your skin helps the outer skin cells stay hydrated by pulling water from deeper skin layers, absorbing moisture from the atmosphere, and by blocking water evaporation through your skin surface. This keeps your outer-surface cells healthy, moist, and supple.

The reason you may not be able to depend entirely on your skin to adequately maintain moisture day in and day out, year after year, is that the skin's natural moisturizing mechanism changes throughout your life and varies from person to person.

Here are some factors that contribute to your skin's natural moisturizing system:

- Your genes. Some people inherently have dry skin, including disorders such as eczema. Others have inherently oily skin, which can result in acne.

- Your age and hormonal status. The production of oil is tied to your hormones. Younger women produce more oil; older women less. After menopause, skin can become very dry because of the steep drop in estrogen.

- The climate you live in. Cold weather, dry air, and windy locales all contribute to dry skin. These climates cause more water evaporation through the skin's surface, and less water is available in the air for your skin to absorb.

- What you do for a living. If you have a job that exposes you to drying chemicals, you are more likely to have dry skin. You also are more likely to be cleansing your skin, especially your hands, three or maybe four times a day. Excessive cleansing, even when necessary, can dry out your skin.

Many people think that applying a topical moisturizer means that they are directly adding water to their skin. That is not true. When you use a topical moisturizer on your skin, basically you are helping your skin retain water by occluding the surface and blocking water evaporation through the skin. Moisturizers do not put water back in the skin directly, but some of the ingredients do help the outer skin cells absorb water from the atmosphere and also from deeper skin layers. The ultimate desired outcome is to increase water in your skin's outer surface cells.

Moisturizers treat and help prevent dry, cracked skin and improve the skin's barrier function, but that's not all. They improve skin tone and texture, giving your skin a healthy, glistening glow. By attracting water, moisturizers also plump up skin cells, creating the appearance and texture of smooth, wrinkle-free skin.

Many different moisturizers line the shelves of skin-care shops, beauty salons, and pharmacies.

Which moisturizer is best for you?

Your Moisturizer

A number of great inexpensive moisturizers can be found at your local pharmacy. Rather than name specific brands, for this chapter and all chapters where I discuss how to choose skin-care products, I suggest you look at the products you currently use and compare them to the ingredients listed. If they don't match up, take your copy of *The Skin Commandments* with you to the store and choose the right product based on your skin type, keeping in mind all you have learned in Skin Commandment II: Honor Thy Skin, where I instruct you to choose products free of fragrances, dyes, and allergenic preservatives.

Choosing
a Moisturizer

Each time you cleanse to remove excess oil and dirt, the next logical step is hydration. Once again, the first rule for any product you apply to your skin is that the product be mild. Look for products free of strong fragrances and brightly colored dyes, and also beware of preservatives that may cause allergies. Moisturizers with these additives all have the potential to cause irritation, and the goal with skin care is to always be gentle.

"Won't any high-priced, designer-label moisturizer do?"

Not necessarily.

And you don't have to have one flown in from Paris, Beverly Hills, a spring in Switzerland, or one derived from an exotic shrub in the Amazon. As with your cleanser, consider your skin type before you choose a product and begin moisturizing. Again, you don't have to spend a lot to get a good product.

Depending on your skin type and the area on your body you are moisturizing, you will want a water-based product—made mostly with water and lighter moisturizing agents—or an oil-based product, which contains heavier, occlusive ingredients designed to prevent water from leaving the skin.

The more oil added to a moisturizer, the thicker and greasier it is—and the more effective it is for dry skin. Also, the more oil in a product, the more likely it is to clog pores and cause acne, especially when used on the face. Water-based products are lighter and contain fewer occlusive ingredients. "Oil-free" products are free of heavy occlusive ingredients, and are usually labeled "non-comedogenic," which means they will not clog your pores.

Moisturizers contain emollients, ingredients that soften skin, make skin more supple, and soothe irritated skin. Moisturizers also contain humectants, the ingredients that attract water. Many moisturizers also mimic the skin's own natural moisturizing system by offering synthetic ceramides, fats, and cholesterol, all essential molecules responsible for skin-cell cohesion that assist your skin in retaining moisture.

How Often
Should I Moisturize?

In Skin Commandment III: Cleanse Correctly, I've instructed you to cleanse your face twice a day if you have normal skin, skin that is neither oily nor dry. For normal skin, the same rule applies to moisturizing. A water-based moisturizer is ideal for normal skin. You want a product that goes on light, not greasy.

Moisturize your skin twice a day immediately after cleansing in the morning and at night. Because you will be applying sunscreen to your face each morning, your sunscreen can act as your morning moisturizer. In the evening, you may use a separate moisturizer that does not contain SPF, perhaps one that includes antioxidants, such as vitamins C or E, CO-Q10, or green tea. (For a list of potent topical antioxidants, see Skin Commandment VI: Fight Free Radicals.)

If you have excessively oily skin, moisturize just once a day in the morning with a sunscreen appropriate for your skin type. Oily skin benefits from oil-free moisturizers and products advertised as non-comedogenic.

For dry skin, moisturize more frequently. Depending on the severity of the dryness, you may want to add two to three applications. For the face, stick to water-based products but increase your frequency of application.

Dry skin on the body calls for an oil-based moisturizer. Products with petrolatum will help treat dry skin on the chest, back, arms, and legs. Also look for humectants like glycerin and urea, which help attract water. Products with lactic acid and glycolic acid help exfoliate the dry, dead skin cells at the same time that they moisturize.

If you have excessively dry skin that cracks in winter or under other harsh conditions, speak with your dermatologist about how to best care for your skin.

Dr. T's Tip for Permeating the Barrier

Your skin works to prevent foreign substances from entering, so in order to help make a topical moisturizer effective, you have to fool your skin into letting in moisture.

Here's the trick: When you get out of the shower or finish cleansing your face, pat your skin lightly with a soft towel so that it remains damp. Apply your moisturizer. The moisturizer will bind to the water molecules on your skin, and together they will be absorbed by your skin cells through tiny channels in your skin called aquaporins to effectively lock in moisture.

Well-hydrated skin appears and feels soft, smooth, moist—slightly dewy.

Keep in mind that there's no guarantee that any moisturizer will live up to all of its advertised claims. Moisturizers are considered cosmetics, so the Food and Drug Administration (FDA) regulates them in a different and more lenient manner than it does drugs. A good moisturizer replenishes your skin's moisture and hydrates your skin cells without irritating your skin or clogging your pores.

The "Natural" Skin-Care Scam

Beware of the term "natural," which is thrown around a lot in skin-care ads. The term implies "better" or even "good," but that is not always the case. In skin care, the term natural is, in fact, completely arbitrary. Tobacco (a plant) and feces (a normal byproduct of metabolism), for example, are both produced naturally. You don't see many people advocating for their use as ingredients in skin-care products just because they are "natural!"

Many natural ingredients are great, but some have no effect on skin at all and may even be harmful, potentially causing damage and irritation. More important than if something is natural is whether it has been studied and scientifically proven to be beneficial to the skin.

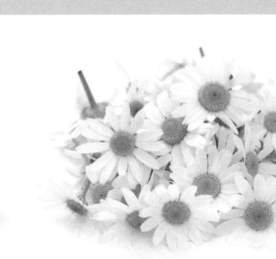

Natural Moisturizers

Below is a list of several natural moisturizers that work great to soothe, soften, and lubricate dry, flaky skin. Additional properties are noted here too, with strong scientific evidence available to validate them. Keep a close watch for any skin reactions, including allergic rashes. I would suggest limiting the use of natural moisturizer to the body—not the face. Because natural moisturizers are typically occlusive, they can clog pores and lead to acne when used on the face. See your dermatologist if you have a troubling reaction.

Aloe vera
Derived from a plant (*Aloe vera*). Anti-inflammatory properties.

Beeswax
Derived from honeycombs. Occlusive properties.

Chamomile
Derived from a flower (*Chamomilla recutita*). Anti-inflammatory and antioxidant properties.

Jojoba
Derived from a waxy seed produced by a shrub (*Buxus chinensis* or *Simmondsia chinensis*). Antibacterial, analgesic, antioxidant, and anti-inflammatory properties.

Shea butter
Derived from the fruit of an African tree (*Butyrospermum parkii*). Anti-inflammatory properties.

Oatmeal

Derived from wild oats (*Avena sativa*).
Anti-inflammatory properties.

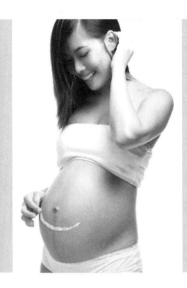

Myth: Cocoa Butter for Stretchmarks

Pregnant women and others who wish to treat or prevent stretch marks commonly use cocoa butter, which is derived from cocoa beans from the tree Theobroma cacao. Numerous studies indicate no change in stretch marks treated with cocoa butter versus other moisturizers.

Moisturizing your abdomen (including stretch marks) during pregnancy does help improve the skin's appearance and texture. You may use cocoa butter if you choose, but any moisturizer will do.

Witch hazel

Derived from plant leaves (*Hamamelis virginiana*). Astringent and exfoliating properties.

Almond oil

(Oleum amygdalae) Derived from the fruit of the almond tree (*Amygdalus communis*). Rich in vitamin E.

Coconut oil

(*Oleum cocos*) Derived from the fruit of the coconut palm (*Cocos nucifera*). Rich in fatty acids.

Evening primrose oil

Derived from seeds of the plant (*Oenothera biennis*).
Rich in fatty acids.

Olive oil

Derived from the fruit of the olive tree (*Olea europaea*). Antioxidant properties. Rich in fatty acids.

Peanut oil

Derived from peanuts (*Arachis hypogaea*). Anti-inflammatory properties.

Safflower oil

Derived from seeds of the safflower plant (*Carthamus tinctorius*). Rich in fatty acids.

Sunflower oil

Derived from seeds of the sunflower plant (*Helianthus annuus*). Rich in fatty acids.

Sesame oil

Derived from seeds of the sesame plant (*Sesamum indicum*). Antioxidant properties. Rch in fatty acids.

All-Purpose Tea Tree Oil

Tea tree oil, which is derived from leaves of the tree species Melaleuca alternifolia, is used commonly for its antiseptic properties in over-the-counter preparations to treat acne, nail fungus, and other rashes.

Although it has proven benefits for mild to moderate forms of acne and has shown slight improvement of nail fungus, tea tree oil is not effective for severe forms of acne, nail fungus, and other rashes. See your dermatologist for more effective treatments and think twice before reaching for tea tree oil for all of your skin maladies.

Hydrating
from Within

Now that you understand the importance of using topical moisturizers to hydrate externally, let's look at how you can boost your beauty by increasing your skin's hydration internally.

Our bodies are made up of 60 percent water—that's how crucial this particular molecule is to our lives. When you drink water, you are providing oxygen and nourishment to your cells by increasing blood flow to your organs, including your skin. When your body is dehydrated, it doesn't function well. When your body doesn't function well, your skin suffers.

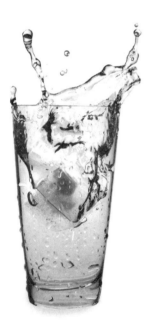

Dry Skin vs. Dehydrated Skin

Many patients ask, "My skin is always dry. Does that mean I'm not drinking enough water?" or "I'm breaking out—does that mean I need to drink more water?"

The answer to both of these questions is no.

Dry skin is due to a lack of moisture in your outer skin layer. Acne is due to overactive oil glands, clogged pores, and bacteria.

Drinking water provides increased blood flow, oxygen, and nourishment to your skin.

HOW MUCH WATER SHOULD YOU DRINK?

Recommendations range from six to twelve glasses of water each day. The Institute of Medicine is in favor of nine cups of beverages a day for women and thirteen cups for men, but that may be excessive for you, depending on your general health.

Dr. T's Tips for Going to the Well

You don't need to carry a giant jug of water by your side at all times. Use common sense.

Here are some simple guidelines for daily water consumption:

– Drink a glass of water when you get up in the morning.

– Drink a glass of water before bed.

– Drink a glass of water every two hours from 8 a.m. to 10 p.m.

– Drink a glass of water before you work out.

– Drink a glass of water after you work out.

– Drink two glasses of water whenever you are thirsty.

Add extra water to your daily routine if your climate, your work environment, or your activity level requires it. You want your water intake to suit your lifestyle.

If you're on the slopes or the deck of a private party boat—and no one is around to test your skin turgor—there are some easily recognizable symptoms of dehydration. If your urine is concentrated and a dark yellow color, your body is telling you to stop what you are doing and drink some water.

"What if I need more flavor than the taste of water?"

There are other options. Juice is mostly water. Of course, most commercially prepared juices also have high sugar and caloric content, so they are not good choices. You may want to make your own juice at home, using fresh fruits or vegetables.

Dr. T's Hydrating Recipes

– *Boil two cups of water and one tablespoon of fresh sliced ginger. Steep for ten minutes on medium heat. Pour mixture into a pitcher of cold distilled water. Add one half cup of cut peppermint stems and one sliced unpeeled cucumber. Chill overnight and enjoy.*

– *In a pitcher, combine one gallon of distilled water, one sliced lemon, one sliced orange, and one half cup of fresh parsley stems. Chill overnight and enjoy.*

– *In a pitcher, combine one gallon of distilled water, one tablespoon of pomegranate juice, one half cup sliced strawberries, and one lime, sliced. Chill overnight and enjoy.*

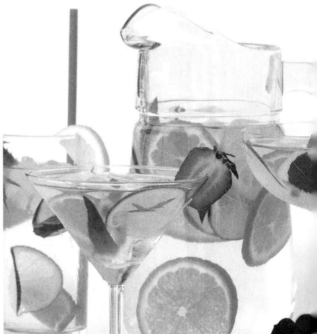

Water from a Coconut

Young coconuts contain a clear liquid called coconut water, long popular in some tropical and temperate parts of the world and now available almost everywhere in cans, cartons, or bottles.

Coconut water is hydrating, tastes great, and is low in sugar and calories. Coconut water also is high in potassium and has the same balance of electrolytes as human blood to the extent that it can safely be infused into the bloodstream. Medics in World War II safely used coconut water intravenously to replace blood volume in combat victims.

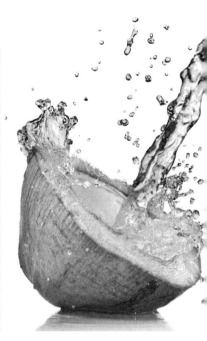

In case you are considering reaching for coffee, tea, or a cola beverage, you need to know that caffeine is a diuretic, which causes your body to lose water. Diet soft drinks offer artificial sweeteners, and few people committed to good nutrition are in favor of artificial sweeteners.

Alcohol also is a diuretic, so don't even think about it.

No way to get around it—drinking water really is the best way to hydrate your body internally. Squeeze some lime or lemon into that glass of water or pour in a splash of pomegranate juice. Figure out how to get more water into your body throughout the day, because staying well hydrated affects the health of your skin, and that definitely affects the beauty of your skin.

WHAT WATER SHOULD YOU DRINK?

Here are some tips:

- Avoid tap water that is high in chloride, lead, and other heavy metals.

- Bottled spring water is not always pure from springs, so do your homework.

- Consider having your water tested and installing a home-purifying system.

- Distilled water is an excellent option—the distillation process removes bacteria, viruses, heavy metals, and other contaminants.

"I've read that drinking alkaline water is best. Is that true?"

That's true for people in the multimillion-dollar industry that promotes alkaline water products. They claim that drinking alkaline water helps remove acid from the body, prevents illness, and slows aging.

However, studies demonstrate that drinking alkalinized water has little or no effect on blood pH, which is under tight regulation by your kidneys and lungs. To date, scientific research has not caught up to the claims made by alkaline water proponents. For now, stay tuned for further studies to validate these claims.

HYDRATING FOODS

We've established that drinking water is the best way to hydrate your body from within, but there are other options. Food also can be a source of water. Surprised?

Tomatoes are about 90 percent water, and watermelons have that name for an obvious reason. What is not obvious at first is that eating the right foods hydrates your body at the cellular level and offers about one-fifth of the water you need each day.

What are those foods? Primarily raw, plant-based foods, healthy foods full of antioxidants, and foods that replenish your body with vitamins and minerals and hydrate your cells at the same time. Increasing your consumption of these foods and other antioxidant-rich foods is key to minimizing the effects of sun damage and aging. (For more on antioxidant-rich foods, see Skin Commandment VI: Fight Free Radicals.)

Dr. T's Hydrating Soup Recipe

Try my favorite antioxidant-packed gazpacho. This water-rich, hydrating dish is packed with vitamins A, C, E, and K; calcium, iron, lycopene, lutein, omega-6s; potassium, and folic acid. It's easy to make and it tastes good, too.

In a blender, combine two cups chopped tomatoes, one cup chopped cucumber (peeled), ½ teaspoon chopped jalapeno pepper, ¼ cup extra virgin olive oil, ⅓ cup fresh lemon juice, ½ teaspoon sea salt. Blend on High and refrigerate mixture for an hour. Before serving, add chopped bell peppers, onions, or avocado slices. This makes four servings. Serve cold.

Refreshing Fruits and Veggies

The best way to remember the fruits and vegetables that help hydrate the skin from within is to think "crisp." Water-rich fresh produce benefits the body in many ways, including hydration. Here are some examples:

– apples

– broccoli

– carrots

– cauliflower

– cucumber

– eggplant

– grapefruit

– jicama

– lettuce

– onion

– spinach

– tomatoes

– watercress

– watermelon

Final Contemplation for Holistic Hydration

Numerous ways to hydrate internally as well as externally are available. Using a moisturizer suited to your skin type, drinking water, and eating raw, water-rich, plant-based foods are the best ways to replenish your body and skin's moisture.

Do all this and your health and skin will always be their best.

SKIN
COMMANDMENT

V

EXFOLIATE EFFECTIVELY

OBEYING SKIN COMMANDMENT V

Exfoliate nightly with a retinoid-based product
based on your skin type.

Perform an at-home mini-peel once a week
on your face and body.

Have a superficial chemical peel performed
once a month at your dermatologist's office.

Use loofah scrubs, shower scrunchies, and soft-bristled
brushes gently on the body and pumice stones
on the hands and feet, but never on the face.

If you waited for an onion to shed its paper-thin skin on its own, how long would it take to make a salad? Just as you actively peel that onion, you can speed up the shedding of old, dry cells from your skin, too.

As I explained earlier, your skin cells grow from deep to superficial, expanding out from the inside. The outer layers of your skin peel off—sort of like a snake's—eventually revealing new, shiny skin underneath.

When you take charge of this process, when you purposely remove that outer layer of cells, the texture of your skin changes much faster—and always for the better.

Exfoliation leaves you with new, smoother, softer, brighter skin. Plus, exfoliation diminishes fine lines and softens deeper lines. Over time, exfoliation evens out skin tone.

Natural skin exfoliation is a slow process. You can't count on it to help you shed old layers of skin—or to reduce blotchiness—in a timely way. To the rescue come a variety of exfoliation treatments in the form of creams, gels, lotions, cleansers, masks, chemical peels, and other procedures.

All these methods hasten cell renewal, and all, over time, will leave you with fresh, radiant, baby-soft skin.

Introducing Retinoids

Any discussion of exfoliation must start with a discussion of retinoids, which are derived from vitamin A. Used in medications, retinoids treat acne, psoriasis, and a variety of other skin disorders. Studies show they may also prevent certain forms of skin cancer.

Used in anti-aging regimens, retinoids increase the rate of exfoliation, promote new skin cells growing to the surface, help repair sun-damaged skin, reduce wrinkles, even out skin tone, and reverse signs of aging.

Your Skin-Care Schedule

You already know that applying sunscreen every day is the most important thing you can do for your skin. The second most important step you can take to achieve healthy, beautiful skin is to apply a topical retinoid every night. The third step is to apply moisturizer according to your skin type.

Here is my recommended schedule for each day:

Morning	Night
1. Cleanse	1. Cleanse
2. Apply a moisturizer with sunscreen	2. Apply a topical retinoid
	3. Apply moisturizer (unless you have oily skin)

"Aren't retinoid products available only by prescription?"

No.

Some retinoid products are available over the counter; others are available by prescription only. Both are good options.

However, over-the-counter products, such as retinol, take much longer to work because the potency of retinoid in the products is far lower. That said, over-the-counter retinoids irritate the skin far less, and studies demonstrate that they are effective. Keep them in mind if you have sensitive skin and budgetary concerns. Look for products with at least 0.5 percent retinol packaged in air-tight, non-transparent packaging that protects the product from sunlight.

There are three main prescription products: tretinoin, tazarotene, and adapalene. Each one, acting in slightly different ways, triggers retinoid receptors, or molecular switches, in skin cells, and each is commonly used to treat acne.

They also will:

- unclog your oil glands and pores

- reduce blotchiness and even out skin tone

- decrease fine lines and wrinkles

- promote collagen synthesis

- promote angiogenesis (new blood vessels)

- remove precancerous growths

The result, over time, is healthy, glowing skin.

NOW LET'S LOOK MORE CLOSELY AT EACH OF THESE MEDICATIONS.

Tretinoin

(known most commonly by the trade name Retin-A) is retinoic acid. Available in liquid, cream, or gel form, tretinoin repeatedly has been proven to diminish fine lines and smooth out superficial wrinkles.

Tazarotene

(also known as Tazorac) is tazarotenic acid, available in gel or cream form. When used to reduce superficial wrinkles, this medication is said to be as effective as tretinoin. The strongest of the three main prescription retinoids, tazarotene is great for people with oily skin.

Adapalene

(also known as Differin) appears to improve photo-damaged skin, but more research is needed. I do recommend it for dry or sensitive skin that cannot handle retinoic acid or tazarotene.

HOW TO USE RETINOIDS

No matter what your skin type, you want to take it slow with these products and only use a small amount each night. Here are some tips to help you safely and effectively use retinoids.

Before you go to bed at night, wash your face. (See Skin Commandment III: Cleanse Correctly.) Next, place a *pea-size drop* of the retinoid product on a clean fingertip and dab a small amount on each region of your face—cheeks, forehead, nose, and chin. A little goes a long way. Apply the medication, spreading it all over your face. Avoid the corners of the eyes, nose, and mouth. Next, apply your usual moisturizer. (See Skin Commandment IV: Hydrate Holistically.)

When you begin, follow this regimen every night. If your face feels too dry or you see too much flakiness, cut back to every second or third night—or add some moisturizer to the pea-size drop of medication.

Expect flaky, slightly irritated skin at first. Once your skin adjusts to the peeling action of the retinoid, the irritation and dryness subsides. Soothe your skin during the waiting period by increasing your use of moisturizers. If you experience an unusually harsh reaction, call your dermatologist.

"If I start using retinoids on Monday, will my wrinkles and sunspots be gone by Saturday?"

Not so fast.

Even though retinoids increase the rate of exfoliation, achieving that healthy glow I spoke of earlier takes time. It may take three to six months before those pesky wrinkles fade and skin tone begins to even out, and a year may pass before the full benefit of using retinoids kicks in.

Words of Caution about Retinoids

Pregnant women and nursing mothers should not use retinoids.

Also, retinoid products, whether prescription or over-the-counter, make your skin more sensitive to ultraviolet rays, so don't skimp on the sunscreen—and always avoid over-exposure to the sun.

In addition to retinoids, many different exfoliating products are on the market, including scrubs, peels, masks, cleansers, soaps, and pads. Some products are used strictly for exfoliation, while others combine exfoliating agents with other skin-care products.

I've already said I am no fan of cleansers or scrubs that contain coarse micro-beads and other mini crystals. I also spoke out in an earlier chapter against using mechanical brushes or scrubbers on the face. All these products may irritate or damage your skin, so please stay away from them.

Loofahs, shower scrunchies, and soft-bristled brushes are good tools for gentle exfoliation elsewhere on the body, but none of these products should ever be used on the face. Pumice stones may be used on the palms and soles. See Skin Commandment II: Honor Thy Skin. For effective exfoliation on the face, stick to the targeted treatments discussed in this chapter.

What's Behind the Mask?

Exfoliating masks are no mystery. These masks exfoliate your skin by sticking to the outer layer of skin and removing dead cells as the mask dries and is peeled off.

Used once or twice a week, a facial mask can remove blackheads and dead cells and soften facial skin. Choose one that suits your skin type and is gentle.

Counting
on Chemistry

Chemical exfoliators—known commonly as chemical peels—also can help turn over and renew your skin cells. Don't be alarmed by the term "chemical." Many of them are derived from fruit. These specifically targeted products can do less harm to your skin than scrubbing away with other so-called "natural" scrubs or home devices.

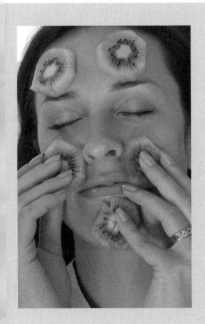

Food on Your Face

This month, the pumpkin facial mask and body scrub is in vogue; next month, it may be the melon mask or apricot scrub. Products also are available that include sea salt, sugar, yogurt, avocado, kiwi—even honey.

Whoa—we're not cooking here! We're not looking to one-up the neighbor's secret Caribbean rub or barbecue marinade. Why put food on your face?

If rejuvenated skin is what you're after, talk to your dermatologist about targeted, effective treatment options. If scientifically proven, naturally derived chemical exfoliants are what you need, see alpha hydroxy acids on the facing page. If natural emollients are your heart's desire, see Skin Commandment IV: Hydrate Holistically.

Let's look at the different types of peels, which are classified according to the type and percent of acid present and the depth of skin penetration. Based on their depth of penetration, chemical peels can be divided into three groups: superficial, medium, and deep.

Superficial chemical peels include alpha hydroxy peels and beta hydroxy peels. Both help you achieve smoother, softer skin, both address fine lines and blotchiness, and both increase penetration of other topical skin-care products such as moisturizers or antioxidant-rich creams. Salicylic acid, the only beta hydroxy acid, is oil-soluble, so it penetrates oily skin more efficiently, which is why it is used in many products that treat acne. Sun-damaged skin responds well to alpha hydroxy acids. These are naturally occurring acids that are derived from foods.

The Acid Lineup

Here is a list of alpha hydroxy acids, with the two most common listed first:

Glycolic acid
Made from sugar cane, glycolic acid peels exfoliate the outermost layer of skin and also stimulate collagen growth

Lactic acid
Derived from sour milk or bilberries

Citric acid
Derived from lemons, oranges, limes, and pineapples

Malic acid
Derived from apples

Tartaric acid
Made from grape extract

Other common superficial peels include low-percentage (10-20 percent) trichloroacetic acid (TCA) peels and Jessner's solution. Jessner's solution, developed by a dermatologist, is a superficial peel made up of salicylic acid, lactic acid, and resorcinol in an ethanol base. Often, patients will have a Jessner's peel before a TCA treatment, to better prepare the skin.

Superficial chemical peels cost anywhere from $40 to $200, depending on the area of skin treated and the concentration of the peeling agent.

Cleansers and moisturizers sold over the counter often contain some of these acids (most commonly salicylic acid, glycolic acid, or lactic acid), and you may choose to use these products as part of your skin-care regimen—but beware of using too much too frequently.

Medium-depth peels include 35 percent TCA peels and combination peels such as TCA with glycolic acid or TCA with Jessner's solution. These peels are used to treat deeper wrinkles, blemishes, and uneven pigmentation.

Your skin type, the depth of your wrinkles, and the extent of sun damage will determine whether a medium-depth peel is best for you. Ask your dermatologist for his or her recommendation. Medium-depth peels range from $500 to $1,000.

Deep peels include the phenol peel, the strongest of the chemical solutions. These are used mainly to treat deep facial wrinkles, blotchy or damaged skin caused by sun exposure, or pre-cancerous growths.

Because the results of deep peels are unpredictable and the procedure is risky—it often requires heart monitoring—I don't recommend deep peels. See Skin Commandment IX: Love Thy Laser for safer, more elegant treatments that I prefer as alternatives to deep chemical peels.

The bottom line:
For all skin types, I recommend performing an at-home mini-peel using either an exfoliating mask or cleanser (read ahead to Dr. T's At-Home Mini-Peel). I also recommend a superficial chemical

peel once a month if the budget will bear it. If your sun damage and wrinkles are significant, speak with your dermatologist about a medium-depth peel or laser procedure.

Most peels typically take about fifteen minutes. First, your face will be thoroughly cleansed, then the chemical solution will be applied. Some patients report a mild tingling or burning sensation. With superficial peels, there is no down time for recovery. Medium-depth peels require a few days of more intense peeling and redness.

"I've got this one blotchy spot on my face. Do I have to get a full peel?" No.

Peels work well for treating the entire face or for isolated trouble spots. Peels also work great on the backs of blotchy, sun-damaged hands.

Always have any chemical peel performed in the office of a board-certified dermatologist. Too often, I have seen patients come in with severe skin reactions, even scars and loss of pigment, from peels done by improperly trained individuals.

DERMABRASION AND MICRODERMABRASION

Dermabrasion and its lighter-weight sibling microdermabrasion are surgical scraping treatments that smooth out skin.

You may be a candidate if you have:

- many fine wrinkles
- precancerous growths
- acne
- deep acne scars
- skin that needs to be cleared of blackheads or debris

Microdermabrasion freshens skin by a process that combines gentle abrasion with suction to remove the outer layer of skin. Dermabrasion, a more aggressive procedure that removes deeper layers, improves scarred skin, and smoothes wrinkles.

Both dermabrasion and microdermabrasion treatments must be performed by a qualified, experienced professional in the office of a board-certified dermatologist. These treatments require specialized, sterile equipment. Treatments take about fifteen to thirty minutes and range in price from $50-$100 for microdermabrasion to $100-$300 for dermabrasion.

Sometimes these treatments are used alone; sometimes they work better with chemical peels or other treatments. Speak with your dermatologist to learn whether you are a good candidate for microdermabrasion or dermabrasion.

Contraindications for Peels

Put off having a chemical peel or dermabrasion or micro-dermabrasion treatments for the following reasons:

– if you have active cold sores

– if you have open facial sores

– if you have had radiation or chemotherapy treatments

– if you have had isotretinoin acne treatment within the last six months

– if you have uncontrolled eczema or severely dry skin

– if you have had a recent sunburn or tan

– if you have a history of scar formation

If you have a history of cold sores, talk to your dermatologist about taking medication beforehand to prevent an outbreak.

Dr. T's At-Home Mini-Peel

Once a week, you can perform a safe, inexpensive mini-peel at home using a common, over-the-counter exfoliating cleanser. If you have dry, cracked skin or skin with open sores, DO NOT perform these mini-peels.

You will need

– a 10 percent glycolic acid cleanser or a 2 percent salicylic acid cleanser

– a clean, open-weave washcloth for the face

– a soft-bristled brush, shower scrunchie, or loofah scrub for the body

Mini Face Peel

Lather your face up with exfoliating cleanser and some warm water. Do not wash the suds off. Instead, allow them to remain on your face for ten to fifteen minutes or as long as you can tolerate. A tingling sensation is good; an overwhelming burning sensation is not. Be careful to not get any cleanser in your eyes.

When time is up, remove the soapy residue from your skin with warm water and the washcloth, using mildly aggressive strokes to loosen dead skin and other debris from your pores. Apply moisturizer immediately after.

Body Peel

Lather up your brush, scrunchie, or loofah with exfoliating cleanser. Brush your body with moderately aggressive stokes. You can be a bit harsher on the body than the face, but don't overdo it. Allow the soapy residue to stay on the skin for ten to fifteen minutes. When time is up, rinse with warm water and apply moisturizer.

Off With the Old,
Out With the New

Exfoliation is a crucial step in optimal skin care, the obvious next step in a regimen that includes cleansing and hydrating. If you resolve to include exfoliation treatments—whether with prescription medications, peels, or procedures conducted at your dermatologist's office—you will be rewarded with brand new skin, again and again.

SKIN VI
COMMANDMENT

FIGHT FREE RADICALS

OBEYING SKIN COMMANDMENT VI

Prevent free radical damage by avoiding UV rays, smoking, alcohol in excess, oxidative foods, and skin-care products with harmful additives.

Increase your consumption of antioxidant-rich foods.

Apply topical antioxidants to your skin separately or as part of your daily skin-care routine in a cleanser, moisturizer, or sunscreen.

Maintaining healthy, beautiful skin requires an understanding of the body's metabolism as well as an effective strategy to combat the factors that contribute to aging and skin cell damage. In the rich and mysterious interplay among every single cell in your body, a constant battle between good and bad forces is at play. The good news is that you can join the resistance.

Ready to arm up and fight for healthy, beautiful skin?

First, you have to know your enemy: ***the oxygen-free radical.***

We need oxygen to live, but it turns out that oxygen also has a dark side. At the molecular level, during normal chemical reactions in your cells, oxygen molecules become electrically charged. These electrically charged molecules are called oxygen-free radicals.

Some free radicals serve beneficial purposes. For instance, the immune system depends on them to help destroy bacteria. But when free radicals are present in excess, they are toxic. They cause damage to your cells' DNA, membranes, proteins, and other vital structures.

This tissue damage is known as oxidative damage. Oxidative damage builds up over time and eventually can contribute to a host of serious diseases, including skin cancer. It is also responsible for many of the visual changes in our skin as we age, such as wrinkles and loose, sagging skin.

In addition to natural processes such as aging, this "radicalization" of oxygen also comes about from exposure to external sources such as:

- UV rays/sun exposure
- tobacco smoke
- excess alcohol consumption
- certain foods
- chemicals in the environment or in your skin-care products

If your body is under siege from free radicals due to sun damage, tobacco smoke, too much alcohol, oxidative foods, additives, or pollutants, your skin will reflect the struggle. We've all seen people whose skin has been ravaged by these unhealthy behaviors, and it's not pretty.

You may volunteer to fight free radicals—or I can draft you. Either way, it's time to arm up.

The Battle Plan

So how do you fight free radicals?

Ever since 1956, when the theory that free radicals contribute to aging was first proposed, scientists have been coming up with ways to prevent free radicals and oxidative damage.

Good news:
Some of those preventive ingredients are found at the grocery store in many common foods you may already enjoy eating. You don't need a prescription—you just need a shopping cart. Others are available in topical skin-care products.

The secret weapon that these foods and topical skin-care products have in common is antioxidants. Antioxidants are chemical substances—vitamins and nutrients that you likely have heard about before—that neutralize free radicals and prevent them from causing further damage.

First, we'll discuss some ways to decrease the formation of free radicals in your body. Next, let's look at the vitamins and nutrients that proudly carry the name "antioxidant" and some specific foods they are found in that will help boost your natural beauty. Then we'll talk about antioxidant-rich topical skin-care products that can help you fight free radicals, as well as enzymes that help repair DNA damage caused by free radicals.

PREVENTION IS ALWAYS KEY

Antioxidants act to counter the effects of free radicals that form due to aging, sun damage, and other external factors. How do you prevent the formation of excess free radicals before they start?

Here's how:
- Never tan. Ever.
- Never smoke. Ever.
- Avoid drinking alcohol excessively.
- Avoid skin-care products with harmful additives.
- Avoid foods that cause oxidative stress.

Ready to look at the details?

First, never tan. Ever.
Although I wrote an entire chapter on the topic of tanning, I feel the need to repeat myself. We know for certain that prolonged exposure of unprotected skin to the sun creates free radicals and damages DNA. Damaged DNA leads to DNA mutations, which lead to skin cancer.

We also know that free radicals from sun exposure damage elastin fibers—your skin's "rubber bands"—and damaged elastin fibers make your skin loose and droopy. Also, UV rays increase free radicals in your skin that directly destroy collagen. In other words, the skin's structural support weakens. The skin appears thin and transparent. Wrinkles check in and refuse to check out.

Read all about it in Skin Commandment I: Thou Shalt Not Tan. Preventing UV damage keeps oxidative skin damage to a minimum, and that preserves your skin's health and beauty.

Second, never smoke. Ever.
Smoking has been shown to increase free radicals and oxidative stress in the skin. A report released in December 2010 by U.S. Surgeon General Regina Benjamin notes that "massive amounts of free radicals in cigarette smoke cause inflammation and oxidative stress, which damages cells, tissues and organs." The report concludes that "there is no safe level of exposure to cigarette smoke."

Go easy on the alcohol.
Like some foods, alcoholic beverages cause oxidative stress by increasing free radicals in your body. They also cause indirect oxidative stress by damaging your liver, which filters free radicals and other toxins. Alcohol harms the liver and impairs your body's internal defense mechanism against free radicals.

Alcohol also reduces the levels of antioxidants in your body and interferes with other important elements and molecules in your bloodstream that participate in the oxidation process. So think twice before you order that second or third drink.

Now, about those skin creams with potentially harmful additives: Topically applied products that contain high levels of allergens can increase free radical damage in your skin. These additives

Avoid This Common Ingredient

One ingredient in particular that should be avoided entirely—unless you have active acne—is benzoyl peroxide, which is particularly highly oxidative.

Too often, patients accustomed to using benzoyl peroxide when they had acne as teenagers continue to use cleansers, pads, or other topical products that include this free-radical-inducing antibiotic.

Prolonged use of benzoyl peroxide results in oxidative injury and accelerated skin aging. Avoid it unless you are using it to treat acne.

literally "rev up" your immune system and recruit inflammatory cells to your skin that act to fight off the offending agent. The immune cells release toxic chemicals—the same chemicals released to fight off bacteria or a virus—and these toxic chemicals increase oxidative stress in your skin. The additives themselves also are directly toxic to skin cells.

For more on this topic, see Skin Commandment II: Honor Thy Skin, which discusses how to choose products free of strong fragrances, allergenic preservatives, brightly colored dyes, and other allergens.

FOODS TO AVOID

Certain foods also contribute to high levels of free radicals in your body. Below is a list of foods that have been shown to increase free radical formation and inflammation in your body. Many of these are processed foods that have been changed from their original form before they reach your table. These "processes" typically include adding some nutrients while removing others and adding preservatives to sustain the "freshness factor" of the food.

Artificial sweeteners
(such as sucralose and aspartame in "diet" products and high-fructose corn syrup in most sodas, sweets, and carbohydrate products)

Refined sugar
(this is common table sugar extracted from sugar cane and stripped of its natural ingredients)

White flour
(found in many cakes, cookies, pastas, white breads, bagels, muffins, pretzels, and crackers)

Hydrogenated oils
(oils with trans-fatty acids, which are added to prolong shelf life, found in margarine and many baked goods)

High-fat foods
(such as ice cream, butter, cheese, chips, most desserts, and red meat)

"Enriched" foods
(foods with artificial vitamins and nutrients added, such as many cereals, breads, pastas, and white rice)

Fried foods
(and foods cooked in oil at high temperatures)

Making better food choices to decrease oxidative stress and inflammation isn't difficult. For instance, switch to raw sugars (such as turbinado), long-acting complex carbohydrate sweeteners (such as brown rice syrup), or natural sweeteners with no potentially harmful synthetic ingredients (such as agave nectar or stevia). Whole-grain carbohydrate products such as oatmeal, brown rice, and flour-less, sprouted breads are easy to find—and tasty, too.

Extra virgin olive oil, a potent free radical scavenger, and non-hydrogenated oils are "good" fats that promote health and beauty. Olive oil, high oleic expeller-pressed sunflower oil, and expeller-pressed safflower oil contain linoleic acid, an omega-6 fatty acid that is crucial for maintaining moisture in the skin. Other sources of good fats are fish, nuts, and avocados, which contain omega-3 fatty acids. Omega-3s exhibit potent anti-inflammatory properties and, like omega-6s, are essential fats for maintaining moisture in skin cells. Grill, steam, or bake when you cook, and look for foods on the menu prepared the same way when dining out.

For optimum nutrition, the zealous prefer to not cook at all, and consume mostly uncooked foods. (See "Eating Raw" in Skin Commandment X: Live Healthy.)

In his best-selling book *The Omnivore's Dilemma*, author Michael Pollan recommends avoiding any food that lists more than five ingredients on the package. He also cautions against eating anything your grandmother has never heard of. He elaborates on these recommendations in his book *Food Rules: An Eater's Manual*, in which he suggests eating fresh, simple food that is free of preservatives and hormones. See Skin Commandment X: Live Healthy for instructions on how to choose produce and meats free of potentially harmful preservatives and hormones.

Who really wants food that is guaranteed to taste okay five years from now?

All of these measures that help prevent oxidative damage—never tanning, never smoking, avoiding excessive alcohol consumption, avoiding harmful creams, and staying away from oxidative foods—will preserve your health, maintain your beauty, and slow down the aging process. How so? Your whole body, including your skin, will be exposed to less inflammation, damage from oxidative stress, and the harmful effects of excessive free radical formation.

GETTING TO KNOW YOUR ANTIOXIDANTS

Unfortunately, regardless of how strictly you adhere to these guidelines, you will inevitably be exposed to free radicals and oxidative reactions that occur due to aging and other normal processes in your body. That's where antioxidants come in to play.

In his book, *Healthy Aging*, Dr. Andrew Weil makes the case for increasing your consumption of antioxidant-rich fruits and veggies to fend off the effects of aging: "... the most practical step we can take to defend ourselves against the ravages of oxidative stress is to *eat more plants*." He emphasizes those last three words because it turns out that the old maxim about eating your vegetables has been proven scientifically true. Plant-based foods contain the most potent antioxidants and free radical scavengers that can help protect your health and preserve your beauty.

Let's focus on plant sources of antioxidants that pertain to the skin. I'll give some examples of common foods that contain them, foods that you can find and easily add to your diet. Many of these antioxidants play a significant role in reducing the effects of UV-induced changes in the skin. Remember, there is no better protection against UV damage than prevention.

Vitamin A

Vitamin A is necessary for repair and maintenance of healthy epithelial cells and is found in food in two forms: Retinol, which is more important as a topical agent, and beta-carotene, which possesses UV-protective capabilities (orange-colored foods such as carrots, sweet potatoes, cantaloupe, squash, apricots, pumpkin, and mangos, and some greens, including spinach and kale). (See Skin Commandment V: Exfoliate Effectively.)

Vitamin C

VItamin C protects collagen and elastin from free radical damage, promotes new collagen synthesis, and contains anti-inflammatory properties (citrus fruits and vegetables).

Vitamin E

Vitamin E protects cell membranes, protects against UV damage and also contains anti-inflammatory properties and immuno-stimulating properties (nuts, especially almonds and hazelnuts).

Supplements for Skin, Hair, and Nails: Do's and Don'ts

Because vitamin A is so crucial in the maintenance and growth of skin cells, a plethora of vitamin A supplements are on the market touting benefits for skin, hair, and nails.

CAUTION: MANY OF THESE SUPPLEMENTS CAN ACTUALLY CAUSE HAIR LOSS AND MAY LEAD TO OTHER, MORE SERIOUS SKIN DISORDERS.

For most people, a plant-based diet rich in red, orange, and leafy vegetables is ideal for obtaining vitamin A. For some people—those who live in sunny climates, those with oily skin, and people with chronic skin disorders such as folliculitis or Grover's disease—vitamin A supplementation may be helpful.

Below is a list of "Do's" and "Don'ts" for skin, hair, and nail supplements. The ingredients in the "Do's" section are helpful for strengthening brittle hair and nails and maintaining skin cell growth and turnover. Most of these ingredients can be found in a daily multivitamin. Speak with your doctor before starting any dietary supplement.

Do's	Don'ts
– vitamin A, plant-derived mixed carotenoids	– mega doses of any of the above ingredients (greater than tolerable upper intake levels—UL) unless specified by your doctor
– biotin	
– gamma-linolenic acid	
– selenium	– animal-derived vitamin A
– zinc	– silica
– iron	– gelatin
– magnesium	– choline
– folic acid	– iodine
– glucosamine	– MSM (methyl sulfonyl methane)

Selenium

Selenium acts as an important component of antioxidant enzymes and also contains anti-inflammatory properties and immuno-stimulating properties (Brazil nuts, walnuts, wheat).

Lycopene

Lycopene possesses UV-protective capabilities (tomatoes, watermelon, guava, papaya, pink grapefruit, red peppers).

Super Foods,
Super Friends

Certain foods, deemed "super foods," are thought to have exceptional free radical–fighting capacity. The following are my favorites because they possess potent antioxidants, they are easily found, and they taste great.

Chocolate and cocoa

Dark chocolate and cocoa powders are filled with antioxidants called flavonoids. Cocoa ranks highest in antioxidant potency among foods that fight free radicals. Remember: Milk chocolate with sugar, caramel, or other high-fat, high-glycemic ingredients don't count. Look for dark chocolate with at least 70 percent cocoa and low sugar content or unsweetened (preferably).

Berries

Acai berries, blackberries, blueberries, raspberries, strawberries—these berries all are loaded with antioxidant plant nutrients called anthocyanidins.

Tea (green or white)

When hot water meets green or white tea leaves, antioxidant polyphenols are released. White tea is made from immature green tea leaves that contain less caffeine.

Pomegranate

This ruby red fruit boasts nearly three times the polyphenols as green tea.

Teamwork Is Key

Antioxidant enzymes are complex proteins—some manufactured in the body and others found in certain foods—that are powerful neutralizers of oxygen-free radicals. In addition to selenium, other important teammates of antioxidant enzymes include CO-enzyme Q10 (CO-Q10), manganese, zinc, and copper, some of which are found in most daily multivitamins.

95

Red wine

The skins of red grapes contain resveratrol, a potent free-radical scavenger. Red wine also contains grapeseed extract. Remember, keep your consumption of red wine to a minimum to avoid counteracting the benefits of red wine with the detrimental effects of excess alcohol consumption. One or two glasses per day are the most you can drink before the bad effects outweigh the good.

If you do not drink alcohol, don't start just so you can benefit from resveratrol. Dietary supplements are available and are a great option. Ideally, it is best to eliminate alcohol consumption altogether and capture the benefits of resveratrol in supplement form.

Wild sockeye salmon

This fish is high in astaxanthin and omega-3 fatty acids.

SOME SEEDS AND SPICES ALSO ARE PACKED WITH ANTIOXIDANTS. AMONG THEM ARE:

Flaxseed

Even a small amount is packed with omega-3 fatty acids.

Chia seeds

Possesses more omega-3s than flax, more antioxidants, and a number of minerals, and has the advantage of easier absorption in the G.I. tract.

Grapeseed

Contains oligomeric proanthocyanidins, a class of flavonoid complexes that, according to some studies, helps stabilize and maintain collagen.

Sunflower seeds

An excellent source of vitamin E.

Pumpkin seeds

Another great source of vitamin E.

Curcumin/turmeric

Contains potent antioxidant properties, anti-inflammatory properties, UV-protective properties, and wound-healing properties.

All of these foods are high in antioxidants. Ideally, you would include these healthy foods in your diet every day, mixing and matching them based on your appetite and culinary interests. Here are some easy ways to get started.

A morning cup of Joe can easily be replaced with a spot of tea, green or white. Instead of a midday snack of chips or candy, look for trail mix at the health food store made with raw nuts, sunflower seeds, flax seeds, pumpkin seeds, or dried berries.

For dessert, rather than indulge in sweets made with high-fructose corn syrup or processed sugars that may actually contribute to free radical formation, opt for one or two small pieces of unsweetened dark chocolate or a bowl of fresh berries.

If you like to decompress at the end of the week with vodka and tonic, pour a glass of red wine instead for a healthy jolt of resveratrol. The zealous, of course, will want to avoid alcohol consumption entirely.

"If I eat salmon and blueberries every day, will it make my wrinkles disappear?" No.

This isn't about getting rid of existing wrinkles. This is about prevention and maintenance. Having antioxidants in your arsenal will prevent damage from free radicals and maintain your beauty. Potentially, over time, using antioxidants may help reverse previous cell damage and reverse some skin changes that are due to aging. For effective wrinkle treatments, see Skin Commandment VII: Thou Shalt Botox, Skin Commandment VIII: Fill 'er Up, and Skin Commandment IX: Love Thy Laser.

Dr. T's Beauty-Full Smoothies

One of my favorite beauty boosters is an antioxidant smoothie brimming with iron, beta-carotene, anthocyanidins, potassium, vitamin A, vitamin E, a host of minerals, and omega-3 fatty acids.

In a blender, place half a bag of raw spinach, ½ cup of fresh blueberries, half a banana, ½ cup almond milk, one teaspoon of chia seeds, and lots of ice. Blend on high until ice is crushed. Serves two.

If you don't like the idea of your smoothie going green (literally), or you want to indulge your sweet tooth in a healthy way, here's another antioxidant-rich shake:

In a blender, combine 1/3 cup pomegranate juice, one banana, and one cup of fresh mixed berries (or a particular berry of your choice). Add ice and blend on high until ice is crushed. Makes one serving.

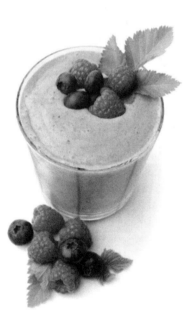

Look at that list of super foods once again. Remember to add them to your diet often. Use these foods, too, to replace foods that contribute to oxidative stress. Over time, as you decrease your intake of foods that contribute to oxidative stress and increase your intake of foods that contain antioxidants, your body as a whole will be healthier. Your cells will have the essential ingredients they need to repair and defend themselves from the effects of aging, sun damage, and daily exposure to environmental pollution, and—that will show on your beautiful, glowing skin.

Dr. T's Must-Have Antioxidant Supplements

When diet is not enough, nutritional antioxidant supplements are available to help you look and feel your best. You don't have to spend a fortune for good vitamins. Here is a basic list of antioxidant supplements I recommend that you take daily. Be sure to speak with your doctor before starting any of these supplements.

– **vitamin C** *(250 mg) (take this twice a day)*

– **vitamin E** *(400 IU mixed tocopherols and tocotrienols)*

– **vitamin D3** *(1000 IU) (Newer studies are recommending higher doses, but the jury is still out. See Skin Commandment I: Thou Shalt Not Tan.)*

– **omega-3 fatty acids** *(2000 mg, molecularly distilled)*

Dr. T's Personal, High-Powered Antioxidant Blend

In addition to the basics, if your budget will bear it, I suggest adding the following high-powered antioxidants that I take daily. Be sure to speak with your doctor before starting any of these supplements.

– *CO-Q10 (200 mg)*

– *alpha-lipoic acid (50 mg)*

– *turmeric (800 mg) (take twice a day)*

– *resveratrol (100 mg)*

– *grapeseed extract (100 mg)*

– *n-acetyl cysteine (600 mg)*

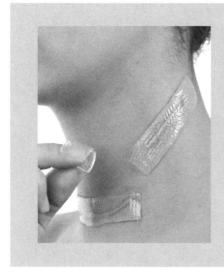

Topical Vitamin E Scar Therapy: Effective?

Many people think that using vitamin E cream will help treat or prevent scars, surgical incision lines, or stretch marks. Numerous studies show instead that vitamin E does not appear to help with any of these conditions.

If you are concerned about scars, your dermatologist will have better options for you, such as cortisone injections, laser treatments, dermabrasion, and silicone patches.

APPLYING ANTIOXIDANTS EXTERNALLY

You can apply some antioxidants directly to your skin. These antioxidant-rich products act to prevent free radical damage the same way as oral antioxidants, but have the advantage of acting directly on your skin cells. However, beware of skin-care products that make false claims. Because the Food and Drug Administration does not regulate cosmeceuticals, many antioxidants on the skin-care market have little to no data to support their use.

Rather than recommend any specific brands, I will focus on topical antioxidants with the greatest data and evidence supporting their use. Look for products that include the following:

Vitamin C

Studies show that topically applied vitamin C boosts collagen production and reduces pigmentation caused by sun damage. Look for products with vitamin C in its ascorbyl palmitate form, a lipid-soluble form that penetrates skin. Vitamin C packaging must be airtight and UV protected so that the vitamin C remains active. Also look for products that combine vitamin C with other antioxidants such as vitamin E, ferulic acid, CO-Q10, and alpha lipoic acid, which all help protect against UV damage.

Vitamin E

Studies suggest that topically applied vitamin E possesses strong protective properties against UV rays, especially when combined with vitamin C.

Ferulic acid

Helps stabilize other antioxidants that fight skin damage. Plus, research suggests that when added to skin creams that contain vitamins C and E, ferulic acid greatly enhances UV protection.

CO-enzyme Q10 (CO-Q10)

An important enzyme cofactor and antioxidant with potent free radical–fighting capacity. Look for CO-Q10's synthetic equivalent Idebenone, which penetrates the skin and has been shown to be effective in topical form at reducing fine lines and wrinkles and also improving skin texture.

Alpha-lipoic acid (ALA)

Because it is soluble in both water and oil, this potent antioxidant is ideal for penetrating skin cells. Some studies suggest that alpha-lipoic acid is effective in preventing some of the visual signs of sun damage and aging and protecting against skin cancer. ALA also has exfoliating properties similar to alpha-hydroxy acids. (See Skin Commandment V: Exfoliate Effectively.)

Green tea

Topical products containing green tea have been shown to protect your skin from UV damage. Due to its anti-inflammatory properties, green tea in creams may improve skin conditions such as rosacea and acne. It also reduces some signs of aging, such as blotchy pigmentation.

Coffee berry

Also known as coffee cherries, this fruit of the coffee plant, long advocated by Native Americans as healthy, is rich in phenolic acids. Scientists first studied the extract because people who pick and harvest coffee cherries have soft, smooth skin on their hands and arms—in spite of being exposed to the blazing sun while working.

Resveratrol

Some studies show that creams featuring this antioxidant prevent UV damage.

Retinol

The second most important topical cosmetic skin-care product after sunscreen. (See Skin Commandment V: Exfoliate Effectively for an in-depth analysis of Retinol.)

Because you will be using sunscreen every morning (see Skin Commandment I), cleansing your skin at least twice a day (see Skin Commandment III), replenishing your skin with moisturizer (see Skin Commandment IV), and exfoliating your skin nightly (see Skin Commandment V), you have plenty of opportunities to apply these enhanced creams to your face and neck in your skin-care regimen. The zealous, of course, may add antioxidant-rich creams as a separate step in skin care.

DNA REPAIR—THE FUTURE OF ANTI-AGING CREAMS

The body has a tremendous ability to repair itself. DNA enzymes repair damage from the effects of oxidative stress due to aging, toxins, UV light, and other external factors.

We know that certain genetic diseases lack these enzymes, which leads to severe skin problems such as premature aging and cancer. There is also strong data that supports that the aging mechanism is attributed to a loss of DNA repair function.

Currently, a number of topical delivery systems are being developed that include some of these DNA repair enzymes. The enzymes—extracted from plants, bacteria, and algae—are packaged into liposomes, a type of cellular membrane, to deliver them directly into the DNA of skin cells, where they act to reverse oxidative damage.

Research continues to determine whether DNA repair enzymes will be beneficial. Stay tuned for more from this exciting field of anti-aging research.

Other reparative ingredients to look for include:

– peptides

– epidermal growth factor (EGF)

– endonucleases

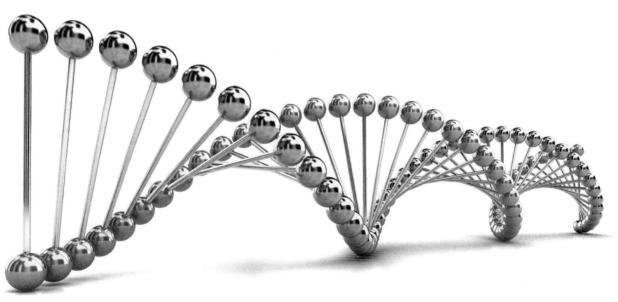

Finalize
Your Battle Plan

Now you know what you need in your armory to fight free radicals: Knowledge of the enemy, ways to prevent oxidative damage, super foods that will help you in the battle against aging, and topical creams and serums that also are standing by as comrades-in-arms.

The science of skin care has come a long way, and the work continues. Studies on natural antioxidants in foods have provided us with guidance about what to eat (and what not to eat). Many scientists now agree that skin-care products enhanced with antioxidants will make great strides in the next decade.

Who stands to win? You—and your skin.

SKIN COMMANDMENT VII

THOU SHALT BOTOX

OBEYING SKIN COMMANDMENT VII

Start getting Botox treatments for forehead wrinkles, crow's feet, and frown lines as soon as you see fine lines when your facial muscles are relaxed.

Choose a doctor specifically trained to provide Botox treatments.

We all know that "botox" is not a verb, but the cosmetic procedure is so popular—more than 5 million people in the United States had treatments in 2010—that people have grabbed this noun and turned it into an action verb.

Got Wrinkles?
Botox 'em!

Botox is short for botulinum toxin and the most popular brand name for this medication (Botox Cosmetic). The same catchy word is now common lingo. Other brand names for botulinum toxin include Dysport, Purtox, and Myobloc. For simplicity, we will use "Botox" to refer to all botulinum toxin treatments because it is the most familiar.

DID YOU SAY "TOXIN?"
Influenced by hyped-up reports in the media, some people worry whether Botox is safe because they have heard or read that it's made from a dangerous, lethal toxin.

IT IS.
If ingested or inhaled, botulinum toxin could kill you. But that has nothing to do with Botox treatments, which are approved by the Food and Drug Administration. Botulinum toxin is a protein produced by the bacterium *Clostridium botulinum*, a bacteria that causes botulism—a fatal, paralyzing infection. Long before it gets anywhere near your face, the toxin is purified. A minuscule, low-concentrated dose is all that is required for effective cosmetic treatments. Over time—three to five months or so—the effects wear off.

Still, maybe you are wondering how I can recommend natural foods to boost your skin's health and beauty in the previous chapter and now I am recommending that you have a known toxin injected into your skin.

Consider this:

Penicillinosis is a potentially fatal fungal infection, caused by the mold *Penicillium*. The discovery that *Penicillium* can fight bacteria led to the development of the antibiotic penicillin—one of medicine's all-time greatest breakthroughs. No one turns up their nose at penicillin because of its humble origins.

Botox's ability to relax muscles has also become a major breakthrough in modern medicine and cosmetic surgery. Originally, botulinum toxin was used by ophthalmologists in the 1980s to treat kids with crossed eyes, a medical condition known as strabismus. Basically, the treatment weakened the muscle that was pulling the eye out of place, leading to proper eye alignment.

One ophthalmologist, Dr. Jean Carruthers, and her husband, Dr. Alastair Carruthers, a dermatologist, noticed that in these same patients, other muscles around the eyes were temporarily paralyzed or weakened, and any wrinkles that had been on the patients' faces were completely gone. Together, they published in 1992 the first study of Botox for the treatment of frown lines.

In 2002, the FDA approved botulinum toxin to improve the appearance of moderate-to-severe frown lines—also known as glabellar lines—between the eyebrows. Now Botox is safely used to treat other facial wrinkles as well.

Multi-Tasking Botox

Botox also is used to treat a variety of medical conditions, including:

– muscle spasms

– excessive blinking

– excessive sweating

– chronic migraine headaches

Feeling comfortable about Botox treatments is easy when you know about its origins in medical science and its long history of safe use. As you can see, Botox is out there doing a lot of good for a lot of people in a lot of ways—and you could be one of them.

Who Benefits from Botox— and When

"I already have forehead wrinkles and I'm only twenty-seven. Am I too young for Botox treatments?"

Not necessarily. I am a big proponent of Botox for a wide range of age groups, and in my practice I recommend early treatment. Basically, Botox prevents facial wrinkles from developing (if you start treatments early) or reduces the severity of wrinkles that have developed (if you start later). So timing is extremely important.

Try this exercise: _____

Take a look in the mirror and smile as wide as you can. Pay close attention to the wrinkles around the outer edges of your eyes.

Now take a look at the horizontal lines on your forehead while your eyebrows are lifted as though you were surprised.

Next, squeeze your eyebrows together tightly as though you were making an angry frown. Note the vertical lines in the center of your brow.

Finally, observe your face while it is completely relaxed, with none of your facial muscles flexed.

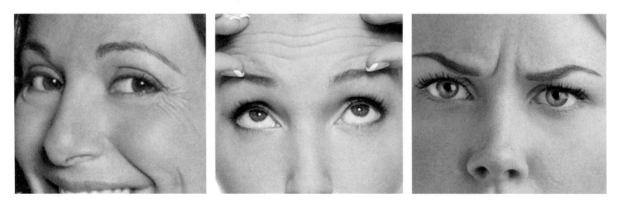

You should consider a Botox treatment as soon as you have fine wrinkles that are present when your facial muscles are at rest, i.e., not flexed.

It is best to treat when the wrinkles are shallow and have not developed into deep, etched-in grooves in your skin. This is assuming, of course, that those wrinkles bother you and you want to do something about them.

If you have fair skin, if you grew up in Florida, if you have a strong brow and find yourself constantly squinting, if you are an actor or model who uses your facial muscles all the time—you may want to start Botox treatments sooner rather than later. In my opinion, your age is not a major factor. Some people see creases and wrinkles in their mid-twenties; some lucky folks make it to forty before their faces begin to show signs of aging.

For every individual, the right time to start treatment is different. I promise you this: The deeper your wrinkles or creases are etched into your skin, the less likely those wrinkles or creases will respond to Botox. So if you want Botox to help you, don't wait too long or you may not be a candidate. If that's the case, your dermatologist will have other recommendations to help improve your appearance, such as chemical peels, lasers, fillers, surgery, or a combination of treatments.

**Botox:
Is It Right for Me?**

Here are some other important considerations for Botox:

– your skin type

– how much sun damage your face has suffered

– how strong your facial muscles are

– how expressive your face is

Here, There,
but Not Everywhere

Say you have a wrinkle that causes you to fret. (Caution: Fretting can cause more wrinkles. See Skin Commandment X: Live Healthy.) You find a qualified purveyor of Botox and make an appointment. You show up, point to your wrinkle, and say, **"Botox it."**

Will you get what you want?
Maybe. Maybe not.

Here's why: ————————————————————————

As I explained, wrinkles on the surface of the skin are due in part to muscle movement below the skin. If a wrinkle has creased the skin, Botox can be used to relax the muscle below, but only if there is a muscle to relax.

Some parts of your face do have muscles immediately below the skin, but other parts have large amounts of subcutaneous fat between the skin and muscle. In spite of its many good points, Botox treatments have no effect on fat. For instance, Botox has no effect on creases in the skin on your cheeks.

You know those crinkly "cigarette paper-like" wrinkles under the eyes? Botox treatments can't help with those either, since those wrinkles are due to loose, redundant skin that may require a laser treatment or surgery. (See Commandment IX: Love Thy Laser.)

If you point to wrinkles on the lower part of your face, such as lines around the mouth, in my opinion the results from Botox treatments alone are modest at best. Botox may need to be combined with other injections or laser treatments to effectively treat wrinkles around the mouth. (See Commandment VIII: Fill 'er Up and Commandment IX: Love Thy Laser.)

Botox at Its Best

Botox works best in the following areas:

– the forehead

– the frown lines between the eyebrows

– the outer part of the eyes, where crow's feet nest

What to Expect at a Treatment

Don't confuse Botox treatments with surgical procedures. Botox is administered by injection. The injections—which take no longer than five to ten minutes—are done with very fine needles. You may feel some light pinching or pressure, but you likely will not feel any real pain. Sometimes, numbing cream or an icepack will be used ahead of time in the area to be treated, but most of the time, no anesthetic is needed.

Before your first treatment, your dermatologist will talk to you about your health history. Expect to be asked about all medications and supplements—prescription and nonprescription—that you take, any allergies you have, and whether you are planning any surgery. If you are pregnant, hope to become pregnant in the near future, or are breast-feeding, you will have to wait to start treatments.

Your dermatologist may look to the Glogau Classification of Photo-aging (named for Dr. Richard Glogau, a clinical professor of dermatology at the University of California at San Francisco) to help determine the extent of wrinkles and photo-aging on your skin. This classification system divides patients into four groups based on skin condition. **Here is a brief summary:**

Type I	Type II	Type III	Type IV
<u>No wrinkles</u>	<u>Wrinkles in motion</u>	<u>Wrinkles at rest</u>	<u>Wrinkles throughout</u>
no need for foundation or makeup	some lines near eyes and mouth, a need for some foundation	some discoloration, visible skin growths, need for heavy foundation	yellow or gray skin color, prior skin cancer, makeup appears caked on and cracks

Some dermatologists just use their eyes to assess the condition of your skin. In any case, if you meet the criteria and pass the tests (none of them are written—I promise), then you and your dermatologist can get serious about using Botox treatments to help improve your appearance.

Botox can cause some rare, temporary side effects, among them: bleeding or bruising, droopy eyebrows or eyelids, localized pain, infection, inflammation, tenderness, swelling, redness, or allergic reactions. The most common is bruising at the injection site, which lasts for a couple of days. Before your treatment, you will want to avoid aspirin, ibuprofen, fish oil, or vitamin E supplements, as they all are likely to thin your blood and contribute to bruising.

The Jack Nicholson Effect

When Botox is injected only in the center of the forehead—but not towards the temple—the outer portions of the eyebrows are pulled way up, creating an overly arched brow, kind of like Jack Nicholson's famous raised eyebrows. Although it works for him, this surprised look may not be the one you have in mind. This side effect occurs most commonly when untrained, non-professionals administer Botox treatments in an incorrect injection pattern along the outer forehead.

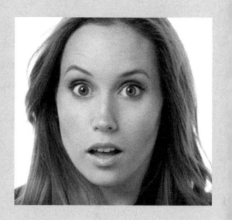

Talk to your dermatologist about any potential side effects that concern you and ask what to do if you experience any of them. After your treatment, be sure to tell your dermatologist immediately if you have any unexpected reactions.

"Will my wrinkles be gone right away?"
Not so fast.

Over the course of three days, the facial muscles that were treated will slowly weaken and become more difficult to move. You should see a noticeable difference in your wrinkles after the first forty-eight hours as your muscles and skin relax.

By day three, the treatment will have taken full effect and your wrinkles will either be gone or significantly diminished. It is important to gauge your expectations appropriately, because not everyone has the same result.

"How much will Botox hurt my wallet?"

The average cost of Botox is about $400 per treatment. Of course, prices often vary, so get that information upfront from your doctor.

Caution: _____

It's good to shop around, but beware of prices that seem abnormally low. This may be a sign that the Botox is significantly diluted or that a non-professional is administering treatments. Because there is an inherent cost for the medication, the price can only go so low—unless something shady is going on behind the scenes.

Quality— Not Quantity—Counts

Many patients ask how many "units" of Botox they need. Some physicians even assign prices per unit. The typical vial of Botox holds one hundred units, so some doctors consider a unit as a dose, and they work under the assumption that most people require ten to twenty units per area. The forehead, the central brow, and crow's feet each are considered one area.

I work differently. This is not about quantity. This is about the art of understanding the anatomy of each patient's facial muscles relative to their wrinkles. To my mind, the number of units is much less important than where the Botox is placed to get the best effect.

Dr. T's Botox Tip

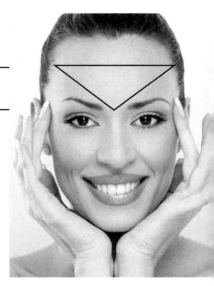

Triangular Tapering Technique.

We all know cosmetic treatment results vary based on the artistic ability of the person performing the procedure. Botox is a perfect example of a procedure where results vary tremendously, ranging from "freakishly frozen" to "the Jack Nicholson Effect" to "rejuvenated and rested."

I employ my own Triangular Tapering Technique, which always results in a perfectly smooth, natural brow.

The Triangular Tapering Technique places more Botox in the upper and central brow and progressively less in the lower and outer portions of the brow in a triangular injection pattern. This ensures that the entire forehead muscle is treated but that the muscles in the outer and lower brow are not as relaxed as the central and upper brow.

The result:

Subtly arched outer eyebrows, no drooping, and certainly no wrinkles.

Too often, injectors make these common mistakes:

– No injection in the outer brow out of fear of causing drooping. This can result in overly arched brows (a.k.a. "the Jack Nicholson Effect").

– Too much injection in the outer brow out of fear of causing overly arched eyebrows. This can result in eyelid drooping.

– Equal injections in the central and lateral brow. This can result in no arching of the brow at all, and flattened eyebrows.

Of course, Botox can also be overdone. We have all seen those faces frozen in time, with skin stretched tightly, faces incapable of registering expression. So I say do—but don't overdo.

What's the best effect?

Getting rid of or softening wrinkles while creating a natural facial expression—one that appears youthful, relaxed, and well rested—that is the intended use for Botox. If your personal goal is to look younger, Botox can do that for most people. We're talking five or even ten, or maybe, in some special cases, fifteen years younger.

Where to Go
for Treatments

Where Not to Go for Botox Treatments:

– a medispa

– a day spa

– a Botox party at someone's house

– a hair or nail salon

– a shop that sells cosmetics

Basically, avoid any place other than a doctor's office.

When you see someone on the street or on television that has a frozen face, asymmetric eyebrows, drooping eyelids, or other bad results from Botox, the treatment was most likely administered by a non-professional. Other reported cases of severe side effects occurred from treatments by non-professionals as well.

Botox injections are medical treatments that require the services of a physician, preferably a board-certified dermatologist or a qualified professional working in a board-certified specialist's office. These physicians have extensive residency training in cosmetic procedures and must fulfill continuing education requirements to stay up to date on the latest treatments.

Doctors, nurses, and other medical personnel who dabble in cosmetic procedures and have not received formal training are not experts in Botox treatments. Also, do not trust facilities where the

116

doctor is "off site" and the facility is simply using that doctor's medical license to allow nurses, medical assistants, non-professionals, or untrained, unsupervised injectors to administer treatments.

How to Find a Botox Doc

Here are some tips to help you find a doctor to speak with about Botox treatments:

– Look for a board-certified dermatologist.

– Make sure that the doctor's office is accredited and licensed.

– At your consultation, ask the doctor about residency training in and experience with Botox. Also ask if the doctor has completed continuing education requirements.

– Not all dermatologists will have the aesthetic sense you are looking for. Ask to see some before and after photos of patients whose skin and wrinkles are similar to yours.

Be sure to choose a doctor you like and trust. To preserve a wrinkle-free appearance, you will need treatments every three to five months, so you will be spending time with your doctor. Comfort level is important.

DON'T TRY THIS AT HOME

When treatments are provided by a medical professional properly trained to inject it, Botox is safe. When you buy something on-line passed off as Botox and try to inject it yourself, that's not safe. Or sane. If that's a corner you are tempted to cut, think how much it will cost when you visit an emergency room to undo the damage you have done.

This should go without saying, but I won't risk it: Do not try do-it-yourself Botox treatments at home.

Relax

Want to take advantage of the number one cosmetic procedure in the world? Botox erases wrinkles by relaxing the muscles that cause them. This safe, effective treatment can help you look years younger in a matter of days. If your wrinkles bother you and you want a rested, more youthful look, an FDA-approved, time-tested treatment is available—a treatment that more than five million people take advantage of each year.

Your wrinkles are just waiting for you to say: "Botox it!"

SKIN COMMANDMENT VIII

FILL 'ER UP

OBEYING SKIN COMMANDMENT VIII

Use filler treatments to treat and prevent smile lines,
grooves under the eyes, sunken-in cheeks,
concave temples, sagging jowls, and thin lips.

Choose a doctor specifically trained
to provide filler treatments.

Losing fat is good, right?
Not always.

Though aging causes some body parts to plump up, as the years go by, the face loses fat and thins out. A youthful face is full, filled with fluid, fat, and water. As we age, the underlying volume of the skin dissolves, leaving us with smile lines, grooves under the eyes, sunken-in cheeks, concave temples, sagging jowls, and thin lips.

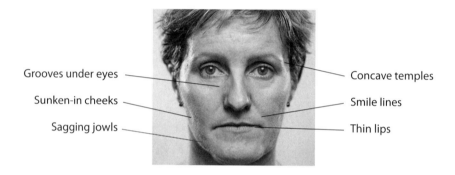

Grooves under eyes — Concave temples
Sunken-in cheeks — Smile lines
Sagging jowls — Thin lips

Don't waste any time mourning these losses. Treatments are available to plump up the skin, refill that lost volume, and restore a beautiful, youthful appearance. Just pull into your local "service station"—a board-certified dermatologist's office—and "fill 'er up."

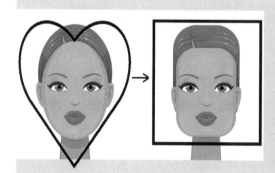

Don't Be a Square

As the face ages, the overall contour progressively changes from heart-shaped (more volume in the upper face that tapers down) to square-shaped (more volume in the lower face as the skin droops). Fillers are used to restore a youthful, heart-shaped face.

In the Introduction, I explained that skin is composed of three layers: the epidermis, the dermis, and subcutaneous fat.

The epidermis is the outer layer of skin. Below is the dermis, composed mainly of collagen, elastic fibers, and other materials that maintain the skin's elasticity. Underneath the dermis is subcutaneous fat—a jelly-like material that gives the skin its plumpness.

If your collagen has dissolved, your elastic fibers have lost their springiness, and your subcutaneous fat has atrophied, you can join the 1.8 million individuals who turned to injectable fillers last year.

These safe and effective restorative treatments may be used to:

- fill in wrinkles
- lift jowls
- rejuvenate thin lips
- erase deep grooves under the eyes
- restore volume in deflated cheeks
- smoothen concave temples
- plump-up thinning skin on the backs of hands

Botox vs. Fillers: What's the Difference?

In Commandment VII: THOU SHALT BOTOX, I recommend Botox treatments to treat frown lines and other wrinkles in the upper face—crow's feet, forehead wrinkles, and frown lines. Botox irons out existing wrinkles and helps prevent the formation of new ones by relaxing the muscles just below the surface of the skin.

Fillers improve facial contours and wrinkles where the skin is sinking or sagging by literally filling them in, especially the smile lines, cheeks, lips, temples, and marionette lines, those puppet-like indentations that appear on either side of the mouth.

Some fillers mimic collagen, subcutaneous fat, or other "inflating" substances naturally found in your skin. Some fillers stimulate your body's own collagen production. In other treatments, fat is moved from one part of the body to the face or the backs of the hands, which also lose their cushiony appearance with time.

Options
at the Filling Station

Liquid Facelift

Most people benefit from both Botox and injectable fillers, a combination often referred to as a liquid facelift, in which the whole face appears plumper, lifted, and rejuvenated—without major surgery.

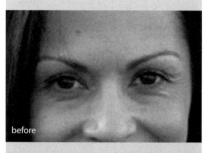
before

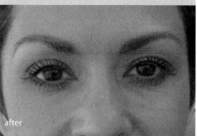
after

procedure by Dr. Nakhla using Botox sixty units total to glabella, crow's feet, and forehead, Radiesse 1.5cc's to cheeks, Juvederm 1cc to tear troughs

A variety of different fillers are available. All of them fill and restore hollow and wrinkled areas of the face and help prevent future sagging. Here are the primary categories of available fillers:

- collagen (Cosmoderm, Cosmoplast, Zyderm, and Zyplast)
- hyaluronic acid (Restylane, Juvederm, and Perlane)
- calcium hydroxylapatite (Radiesse)
- poly-L-lactic acid (Sculptra)
- polymethylmethacrylate (Artefill)
- silicone
- fat transfer (uses your own body fat)

Collagen was the first filler substance injected into the skin. In use since 1981, collagen fillers once were very popular, though some collagen treatments require allergy testing in advance. Collagen fillers include Cosmoderm, Cosmoplast, Zyderm, and Zyplast. Treatments may last three months or longer and cost $400 to $600. Newer fillers that last much longer are now available.

The most popular fillers are made from hyaluronic acid, a natural substance normally found in the skin. Trade names include Restylane, Juvederm, and Perlane. Once in place, these fillers recruit water to the treated area and help the skin retain water. They work best to redefine and plump the lips, to treat superficial wrinkles around the mouth, and to fill in the grooves under the eyes known as "tear troughs." These fillers also may be used in combination with Botox to treat deep frown lines.

Depending on where they are used on the face, most hyaluronic acid fillers last from six months to one year and cost anywhere from $500 to $850 per syringe. You may require more than one syringe depending on the desired effect in the area being treated.

Un-Groovy Grooves

As we age, tissue below the eyes may sink in, causing grooves to form below the eyes, giving the appearance of deep, tired circles. In dermatology, these grooves are known as tear troughs and palpebromalar grooves.

At one time, cosmetic surgeons routinely turned to the knife to remove the baggy fat above the tear troughs. Often, the surgery flattened the lower eyelids and restored a rejuvenated, rested look, but this invasive, expensive surgery also can create an even more hollowed-out appearance. Unless the fat severely protrudes, this surgery may not be necessary.

Today, fillers can make short work of these grooves and restore a rested, youthful appearance to the eyes.

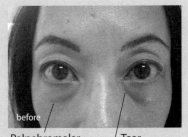

before

Palpebromalar groove / Tear trough

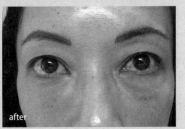

after

procedure by Dr. Nakhla using 3cc's of Juvederm to bilateral tear troughs and palpebromalar grooves

The calcium hydroxylapatite–based filler—Radiesse—is thicker and more viscous than hyaluronic acid fillers. It is used to smooth out the contours of deeper creases, including smile lines, marionette lines around the mouth, divots in the cheeks, and sagging jowls. It works wonders on the backs of the hands where a "skin-on-bone" appearance can occur due to thin skin. It also can create or enhance high cheekbone definition as an alternative to cheek implants.

Radiesse, which can last twelve to eighteen months, costs anywhere from $750 to $950 per syringe, depending on where the filler is injected. Again, you may require more than one syringe depending on the desired effect in the area being treated.

Radiesse also is a collagen stimulator that allows your body to produce new collagen, something the product has in common with Sculptra (poly-L-lactic acid). Sculptra, which is technically not a filler because the effects are gradual, is a powdered form of suture material (the kind of stitches that dissolve) that possesses collagen stimulatory effects. When mixed with sterile water and injected into the face, the collagen-stimulating crystals go to work, and after about three to four weeks, the increased facial volume begins to be visible.

Reinforcing the Skin's Structure

Collagen serves as scaffolding for the skin, and when collagen breaks down, hollows appear and skin volume is reduced. Fillers known as collagen stimulators gradually encourage the growth of new collagen below the skin by stimulating fibroblasts, cells that synthesize collagen, and also by providing structure for that growth.

A few weeks after a treatment, as the product takes effect, the skin begins to fill out once again as the underlying tissue expands.

Sculptra works especially well in the cheeks, the jowls, and where the skin above the temples thins out. Sculptra requires a series of three to six treatments over four months or so, but the increased volume in the skin can last up to two years. Treatments cost $800 to $1,000 per vial. Usually one or two vials are used per treatment session.

A few permanent fillers, including Artefill (polymethylmethacrylate) and silicone, are available, but because the contours of the face continue to change as you age, I don't recommend them. Also, if you don't like the results of a permanent treatment, you are stuck with it—it's a done deal and there's no turning back.

Sometimes, people develop granulomas—disfiguring nodules that form under the skin—after permanent filler injections, even years after the treatment. These granulomas are a sign that your immune system is fighting off a foreign substance. Granulomas also occur with Sculptra injections, though now less commonly with newer injection techniques.

Fat transfer—a procedure that transfers subcutaneous fat from elsewhere on your body to your face or the back of your hands—results in a natural look because, well, it's the real thing. Fat transfer requires liposuction to extract the fat, which is then injected into the cheeks, under the eyes, backs of hands, or lips—the four areas where it works best. Fat transfers in the United States increased by 14 percent in 2010, which speaks to the growing popularity of the treatment.

Philtral column

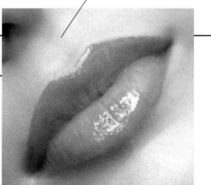

Dr. T's Tips for Luscious Lips

Deep Filling, Medio-Lateral Tapering, and Vertical Lip Columns: Based on the artistry of the injector performing your procedure, the results of injectable fillers in the lips range from "Daffy Duck" to "sexy yet subtle." Here is my advice: If you've never had big lips, you shouldn't try to achieve big lips. The key with lip fillers is to provide shape, volume, and definition to deflated lips, always keeping in mind the individual's natural look and genetics.

I use a deep-filling technique to avoid abnormal lip protrusion, as well as a medio-lateral tapering of filler injection, similar to my technique for Botox. This technique places more filler in the central portions of the lip where most of the lip shaping is needed and less in the outer lip, preventing the duck-like lips you see in someone who has had a botched procedure. I also always address the vertical lip columns in the center of the lip—known as philtral columns—that flatten out and lose definition over time.

Some surgeons report permanent correction with fat transfer, although studies show that when injected in the face, transferred fat lasts up to twelve months. Again, with fat transfer the result is more natural looking than with some other fillers, but other treatments require less effort and less down time and are much less expensive. With fat transfer, you also will pay for liposuction, which may run anywhere from $1,500 to $5,000.

Dr. T's Favorite Filler Combos

Layering Technique: No single filler is perfect for every area of the face and for re-volumizing every layer of skin. Some fillers work best in deeper layers, while others work best injected more superficially. Too often, inexperienced injectors use one type of filler to correct multiple layers of deflated skin, resulting in flattened contours and "monkey-like" faces. I use a layering technique of various fillers for most areas of deflated skin.

Based on my experience, here are my recommendations:

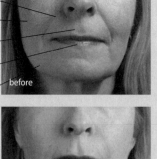

Smile lines
Concave cheeks
Philtral column
Lips
before
Jowls

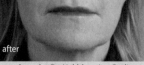

after

procedures by Dr. Nakhla using Radiesse 1.5 cc's to smile lines, Juvederm 1 cc to lips and philtral columns, Scupltra 2 vials to cheeks and jowls

– smile lines: *Radiesse*

– lips: *Juvederm*

– concave (hollow) cheeks: *Sculptra*

– jowls: *Combination therapy with Sculptra and Radiesse*

– tear troughs: *Juvederm*

– concave (hollow) temples: *Sculptra*

– cheekbone enhancement: *Radiesse*

– cheek wrinkles: *Combination therapy with Sculptra, Radiesse, and Juvederm*

– marionette lines: *Combination therapy with Sculptra, Radiesse, and Juvederm*

The Vampire Facelift

Selphyl, a new injectable filler system known as the Vampire Facelift, uses the patient's own blood to make skin look plumper and younger. First, blood is withdrawn and mixed with another substance that separates platelets and fibrin (substances in the blood that are known to stimulate collagen growth), which are then re-injected into the area being treated.

A few weeks after treatment, the face is said to fill out as collagen production increases. Treatments are expected to last up to fifteen months. The cost is $1,200 to $1,600. The jury is still out on the safety and efficacy of this new treatment.

What to Expect at Your Appointment

Filler treatments are fast and practically painless, but that's no reason to pop in at a medispa on a whim. Make an appointment with a board-certified dermatologist with training and experience using fillers. Always ask to see before and after photos of procedures performed by the doctor you are consulting with. That way, you know you are working with someone who understands what treatment to use and how and where to inject the filler.

The entire procedure takes between fifteen and thirty minutes. Before the filler is injected, the area of your face to be treated will be numbed with either a topical medication or an injection of lidocaine, a common local anesthetic.

When the filler is injected, you may feel a pinch or slight pressure. Later, the injection site may be slightly tender, bruised, or swollen. All of these potential side effects go away within a few days and there is no down time afterward.

Where Not to Go for Filler Treatments:

– a medispa

– a day spa

– a filler party at someone's house

– a hair or nail salon

– a shop that sells cosmetics

Filler injections require even more artistry than Botox injections. A botched filler treatment may result in permanent, disfiguring damage, so play it safe.

Filler Finale

Remember how you looked fifteen years ago? Bringing back the apples in your cheeks, a plumper, fuller face—that's where fillers excel. A number of safe, FDA-approved products are on the market, and new fillers are being developed all the time.

Don't wait: Re-inflate and fill 'er up.

SKIN
COMMANDMENT
IX

LOVE THY LASER

OBEYING SKIN COMMANDMENT IX

Use laser treatments to treat blotchy pigmentation, redness in the cheeks, broken blood vessels, and acne scars.

Use laser treatments in combination with Botox and/or fillers to treat deeper wrinkles.

Find a doctor specifically trained in laser treatments.

Every day, patients come in to my office, point to areas on their faces that they wish to improve or blemishes they wish to be rid of, and say, "Hey Doc, can you laser this?"

Multi-purpose Lasers

Developed in the 1940s, lasers are used in medicine, dentistry, manufacturing, and other areas of industry.

In addition to improving the appearance of skin, lasers also are used for tattoo removal, hair removal, and to remove some skin cancers.

Technically, I can't "laser" anything, because the term is not a verb. LASER stands for Light Amplification by Stimulated Emission of Radiation.

Whoa—Nerd Alert! Let me try that again in English.

Put simply, a laser is a specific type of light beam that is used to improve the skin's appearance. However—unlike on *Star Trek*—lasers are not magic wands. They have specific functions, and different types of lasers are used for various applications.

Can I use a laser—or, more correctly, "lase" the skin—to improve skin tone and texture; get rid of skin blotches, red spots, broken blood vessels, fine lines, or deep wrinkles; and restore a more youthful appearance?

Sure. I can do that.

Laser treatments can improve the following conditions:

- skin with blotchy pigmentation

- skin with persistent redness or broken blood vessels

- skin with acne scars

- skin with fine lines and deep wrinkles

130

How do lasers work?

They emit powerful beams of light that pass through the top layers of skin to target problem areas. As the targeted areas (such as bright red blood vessels or blotchy sunspots) absorb the light, the beams are converted to heat. The heat causes the undesired target to disintegrate, leaving you with clear skin.

The same is true for laser skin resurfacing procedures, which are used to treat pitted acne scars, deep wrinkles, and more extreme pigmentation problems. These lasers vaporize and peel off the outer layers of skin.

Let's look at the types of skin problems that are treatable with lasers one at a time, because each requires a specific laser that works a little differently. For simplicity, the various technologies and names of different lasers will not be listed. Speak with your dermatologist to find out which laser is right for you.

The Laser Treatment Menu

BLOTCHY, RED SKIN AND BLOOD VESSELS

Lasers do the best job of removing red blotches and broken blood vessels from the skin. The light beams are absorbed by hemoglobin, a molecule in your red blood cells. The light turns to heat and selectively obliterates the blood vessel, leaving surrounding skin unharmed.

Lasers also work well for ruddiness caused by sun damage or rosacea, which is a chronic skin disease that causes inflamed skin. With rosacea, the forehead, cheeks, chin, and nose appear rosy or flushed due to dilated blood vessels in those areas.

Grandpa's Nose

In extreme forms, especially in men who drink excessive amounts of alcohol, rosacea can cause a "rhinoceros-like" enlargement of the nose, called rhinophyma. We've all seen these gentlemen with bright red faces and puffed-up noses, sipping whiskey at a local pub or family gathering.

Here's the good news: If one of them is your grandpa or pal, make an appointment for him to see a dermatologist, as a laser procedure often can restore the nose to its original shape and color.

See those broken capillaries around your nose and chin? Lasers instantly vaporize those bothersome blood vessels. Tiny, round red moles known as cherry angiomas, also a sign of sun damage, are yet another source of redness that easily can be zapped with lasers.

Arachnophobia

Some people fear spiders; others fear spider veins, small dilated blood vessels near the surface of the skin that can develop anywhere but are common on the legs and face around the nose, cheeks, and chin. These tiny veins, technically known as telangiectasias, got their popular name because they resemble spiders' legs—and that's much easier to pronounce.

Lasers work well for spider veins on the face. Spider veins on the legs respond better to sclerotherapy, a treatment in which a medication is injected directly into the veins to make them dissolve. Sclerotherapy costs about $200 to $300 per session, and usually three to five sessions are needed.

BLOTCHY, BROWN SKIN

Uneven pigmentation due to sunspots (also known as age spots or liver spots) or melasma (pigmentation that occurs most commonly on women's faces due to hormones)— respond well to treatment with lasers.

More on Melasma

Mottled, discolored skin is due to uneven pigmentation below the skin's surface. Most often, the discoloration is due to sun exposure from years past or another condition known as melasma, which can occur during pregnancy, in women taking oral contraceptives, and with certain other medications.

Most of this extra pigmentation shows up on the cheeks, forehead, upper lip, nose, and chin. Melasma is the single most difficult cosmetic dermatologic problem to treat and a common cause of frustration for dermatologists and patients because no one treatment works effectively.

The best treatment is combination therapy—lasers along with diligent use of sunscreen, sun avoidance, and effective exfoliation. (See Skin Commandment I: Thou Shalt Not Tan and Skin Commandment V: Exfoliate Effectively.) Some prescription and non-prescription products also help fade dark spots. Read ahead to next page: Bleaching Creams Don't Actually Bleach.

These lasers target melanin, the pigment found in skin. Beams of light from the laser are absorbed by the melanin, which heats up. The heat causes the dark pigment particles to break up. The dark spots then either peel off or are removed by the immune system.

Bleaching Creams Don't Actually Bleach

"Can't I just use a cream to bleach my dark spots or melasma?"

Not really. But there are topical products that can help. These so-called "bleaching" creams don't actually bleach the problematic pigment the way you might expect them to. Instead, they work by blocking the production of new melanin pigment from your melanocytes—the skin's pigment-producing cells.

This prevents new pigment from forming and gives your skin a chance to renew itself and exfoliate the old, blotchy skin, though it may take several months after starting to use bleaching creams before a difference is visible. Examples of topical skin-lightening products include hydroquinone, azelaic acid, and kojic acid. Ask your dermatologist if one of these products is right for you.

Laser treatments that address pesky pigment issues or bothersome blood vessels take about fifteen to twenty minutes and cost about $250 per session. For the best outcome, usually three to five treatments are needed. There is no down time afterward other than mild, temporary redness. Sometimes the target area may darken and become more noticeable at first, before fading away. Topical numbing medicines are used to reduce discomfort with any of these procedures and pain medicines, and sedatives are not required.

Shining a Different Light

Intense pulsed light (IPL), also known as the "photofacial" (a type of facial that uses light energy), is another way to treat blotchy pigmentation and red spots. Lamps, rather than lasers, are used to discharge high-intensity light that goes after uneven pigment splotches and redness caused by broken blood vessels.

IPL treatments are not as precise as laser treatments, but they generally cost less and can be used to treat both pigment problems and blood vessels during the same treatment. There is good data that shows IPL treatments also stimulate collagen and help with fine lines. Again, there is no down time other than mild redness and slight peeling.

Treatments range from $200 to $300 per session. For maximum effect, you may need three to five treatments and quarterly maintenance treatments.

SMOOTHING THE SKIN SURFACE

Have you ever had your driveway resurfaced?

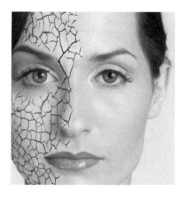

If so, you remember that the top layer of cracked asphalt was removed to make way for a fresh, new top layer. Skin resurfacing is kind of like that, only it's a more precise, more elegant procedure that relies on the natural healing process of cellular renewal.

These treatments, known as laser skin resurfacing, work best on "etched-in wrinkles" such as smoker's lines around the mouth and other deep wrinkles that are not treatable with Botox and/or fillers. Laser resurfacing also works wonders on pitted acne scars and sun-damaged skin with blotchy pigmentation that is too advanced for other procedures.

135

While other lasers emit light in a single beam, the latest skin resurfacing lasers (also known as "fractionated" lasers) send out pulses of light divided into multiple micro beams that leave tiny areas of space in between each target. This technique allows for faster healing and deeper penetration, and it reduces the risk of complications.

In this procedure, water within the skin is the target that absorbs the micro beams of light from these lasers. Again, the light converts to heat, the water temperature in the cells rises, and a controlled burn takes place, causing minimal heat damage to surrounding tissue.

Over time, the old skin peels, and during the healing process— a week to ten days—the old skin is replaced by soft, new, baby-like skin. Although the skin surface appears completely healed, the healing process continues below the surface for months as new collagen formation—known as neocollagenesis—occurs, providing you with progressively enhanced results after six to eight months.

Laser resurfacing treatments take about one hour. Some patients opt for a mild oral sedative or pain medication in addition to the topical numbing cream applied to the face. Laser resurfacing costs between $1,500 and $3,000 for an aggressive procedure. Less aggressive versions cost between $700 and $1,000.

Laser treatments for wrinkles work best when used in combination with Botox and fillers.

CARING FOR YOUR SKIN AFTER RESURFACING

When you get the driveway done, you have to block it off and keep people away for a couple of days. After a skin-resurfacing treatment, you will have to protect your skin.

The doctor will coat your skin with a soothing ointment after the procedure and direct you to use icepacks and sleep with your head propped up to control swelling. Your skin may develop a crust on the treated areas. Leave it alone—that's part of the healing and skin-renewal process. Your skin will peel when it's ready.

You may glow a bright pink at first, and it's not a good idea to apply heavy makeup to the healing area right away. Wait about a week to ten days. In the meantime, you must wear sunscreen. The last thing you want is UV rays from the sun harming your tender, new skin.

The effects of laser resurfacing are considered permanent, but as you age, new occurrences of dark pigmentation or wrinkles may call for additional treatment.

BUYER BEWARE

Without question, laser skin procedures require the services of an experienced, board-certified dermatologist or a qualified professional working in a board-certified specialist's office under supervision. Lasers are safe in the hands of the right person, and downright dangerous in the hands of the wrong one.

Most of the patients I see who have experienced complications—scarring, for instance—with laser treatments had those treatments at medispas or day spas, where poorly trained or even untrained non-professionals perform these complex procedures.

Don't make a bad decision based on a whim, your budget, convenience, or even a friend's recommendation. If you're interested in a laser treatment of any kind, make an appointment with a board-certified dermatologist.

Tighten Up

If what you have in mind is firmer skin around the eyelids, the jowls, and the neck, laser skin-tightening treatments are available that use advanced radio-frequency technology, rather than light, to heat layers of collagen deep below the surface of the skin.

These laser treatments are acceptable for correction of mildly loose skin, and the results are very subtle. If you need more than mild correction, you may want to investigate eyelid surgery, a facelift, or a neck lift, which are still considered the best treatments for severely loose, sagging skin.

Let There
Be Light

Laser technology has introduced new options for individuals who want to restore their appearance without undergoing invasive surgery. These treatments are increasingly popular, remarkably effective, and—in the hands of a trained professional—very safe.

New technology and new uses for lasers in skin care are being developed each day. If skin discoloration, broken blood vessels, deep wrinkles, or acne scars trouble you, then you, too, can learn to Love Thy Laser.

SKIN
COMMANDMENT

LIVE HEALTHY

OBEYING SKIN COMMANDMENT X

For healthy, beautiful skin,
tend to your body, mind, and spirit.

Where does a pimple-popping, Botox-injecting, LASER-slinging dermatologist get off preaching about healthy living, diet, and lifestyle modification?

Here's how:
Changes on the skin's surface are often the earliest indications of major internal dysfunctions. "Seinfeld" jokes aside, dermatologists save lives on a daily basis and are at the forefront of healthy living and wellness.

For example, did you know:

- An itchy rash may be a sign of a vitamin or mineral deficiency.

- Cystic acne or excess hair growth in women may be clues to malfunctioning ovaries.

- Yellowing skin may indicate liver disease.

- Dark pigmentation under the armpits may be a sign of diabetes.

- Hair loss may be due to iron deficiency.

- Sunburn may be a sign of lupus, a multi-organ disease.

Skin changes due to lifestyle behaviors may be even easier to spot. That's because your skin advertises the state of your health to one and all. **For instance, your skin may show signs of:**

- poor nutrition
- dehydration
- smoking
- alcoholism
- high cholesterol
- exposure to environmental toxins
- stress

The list goes on and on. In fact, volumes have been written about the skin changes that occur in an unhealthy, malfunctioning body. Yet all too often, people wishing to improve their skin focus on just that one organ, and do little to improve their general health. These folks—and sometimes their dermatologists—are so focused on the trees that they miss the forest.

Here's the bottom line:

Your body is not the sum of individual organs working alone. It is a complex, interconnected, marvelous machine with harmoniously functioning parts, of which your skin is one. Your skin tells the story of your days in the sun, but it also reflects the general health of your internal organs and your entire body as a whole.

It's no surprise then that healthy, radiant skin that seems to glow from within, is the reward for healthy living. When you stray too far from living healthy, your skin may look dull, your face may appear tired, your overall demeanor may be a little "off," and you may not look or feel quite like yourself.

BAD FOR YOUR BODY, BAD FOR YOUR SKIN

First things first. If you believe that living healthy is best and you want to boost and preserve your beauty, then avoid excess alcohol consumption, don't smoke, and say no to drugs. Those are no-brainers.

As you read in Skin Commandment VI: Fight Free Radicals, these behaviors cause oxidative stress by increasing free radical damage in your body and skin. Drugs and alcohol also harm the liver and impair your body's internal defense mechanism against free radicals.

Wrinkly Facial Expressions

You've seen the wrinkles caused by smoking—deep, vertical lip lines from tightly puckered lips often gripped around a stogie. Almost always permanent, these types of wrinkles are easily avoidable. Don't smoke.

Other facial expressions and emotions to avoid include frowning, furrowing, fretting, squinting, stressing, and scowling. (See "Stressed-Out Skin" ahead.)

Some wrinkles and folds become characteristic of our personal expressions—nothing wrong with that. Smiling is another motion that progressively wrinkles skin. But I won't advise you to quit that.

To sum up, gorgeous skin is unattainable if you are a smoker, binge drinker, or dabbler in illicit drugs. If bettering your body and improving your skin is your goal, then quit smoking, limit your alcohol intake, and stay away from drugs altogether.

DIET AND SKIN

In Skin Commandment VI: Fight Free Radicals, I discuss the harmful effects of free radicals, I encourage you to increase your consumption of antioxidant-rich foods, and I advise you to avoid foods that cause oxidative stress. Again, every organ in your body is affected by what you eat and drink, so you want to make good choices.

Specific suggestions to help you make better food choices are outlined in Skin Commandment VI, but here is the boiled-down version, so to speak, of my recommendations: Fill your plate primarily with whole-grain carbohydrates, fresh raw vegetables and fruits, and lean protein, preferably fish or plant-based sources.

Staying away from foods that cause oxidative stress preserves your health, maintains your beauty, and slows down the aging process by limiting your exposure to the harmful effects of excessive free radical formation.

To recap, foods that have been shown to increase formation of free radicals and oxidative stress include:

- artificial sweeteners
- refined sugar
- white flour
- hydrogenated oils
- high-fat foods
- "enriched" foods
- fried foods and foods cooked in oil at high temperatures

Pinpointing Foods that Cause Acne

Some 40 to 50 million Americans have acne, and it's anyone's guess how many people believe that fried food, greasy food, pizza, and sweets all cause acne.

Ordinarily, they don't—though they may in you.

Huh?

Most large studies have been unable to consistently prove that these common food culprits cause acne. That said, dermatologists all over the world agree that on an individual basis, certain foods do trigger acne in certain patients. For example, if you notice that every time you eat French fries, you break out with zits, stop eating French fries.

Listen to your body. It's that simple.

It is a good idea to wash your face after tucking into greasy foods like pizza or tacos, just to clear away any oil left around the mouth and prevent clogged pores. It's a better idea to avoid these oxidative foods altogether.

If you have acne or acne-prone skin, another food category to limit or avoid is dairy, which according to several studies, has been closely linked to acne. (Read ahead: Dairy Products and Acne.)

Dairy Products and Acne

For decades, dermatologists maintained the notion that acne is unaffected by diet, including dairy products. Today, several studies indicate that the link between acne and dairy consumption is valid. One study published in the *Journal of the American Academy of Dermatology* in February 2005 linked acne to milk (skim), sherbet, cheese, and other dairy products. This is most likely due to the stimulatory effects of hormones in dairy products on oil gland secretion, which is the root cause of acne, although further research is needed to understand the exact mechanism.

Here's my advice. If you have acne or acne-prone skin, switch to soy, almond, or rice milk and avoid dairy products entirely, supplementing your diet accordingly with other sources of calcium, vitamin D, and protein. If dairy products are your palate's delight, at least switch to organically farmed, hormone-free products and limit your consumption to only a few servings per week, although even these products contain the normal hormones found in cow's milk that may contribute to acne.

For optimum health and beauty, I am a proponent of organic produce. There is good data to support the increased levels of antioxidants and nutrients in organically grown fruits and vegetables.

In April 2009, results from Quality Low Input Food (QLIF), a five-year integrated study funded by the European Commission, showed that organic food production methods resulted in higher levels of nutritionally desirable compounds (vitamins/antioxidants and polyunsaturated fatty acids such as omega-3s) and lower levels of nutritionally undesirable compounds (heavy metals and pesticide residues).

Another study published late in 2010 conducted by Washington State University at commercial farms in California suggests that organic strawberries have higher levels of antioxidants and vitamin C than conventionally grown strawberries. A ten-year study conducted by the University of California at Davis indicates that organic tomatoes have measurably higher levels of antioxidants such as quercetin and kaempferol.

Also, in decreasing your overall oxidative stress load, organic produce that has not been sprayed with toxic pesticides is certainly more favorable than produce that has been exposed to such farming methods. If your budget is a major concern, at least make sure the "thin-skinned" produce you buy is organic.

I'm talking about:

- berries
- apples
- leafy vegetables
- tomatoes
- grapes

Excessively Rosy Glow

Some foods—especially hot liquids, alcoholic beverages, and spicy dishes—can trigger rosacea, which is common in women and people with fair skin. The National Rosacea Society lists these possible triggers: _____

- avocados
- cheese
- chocolate
- cinnamon
- citrus fruit
- eggplant
- mint
- sour cream
- soy sauce
- spinach
- vanilla
- vinegar
- yogurt

Monitor whether these foods cause rosacea outbreaks in your skin and change your diet accordingly.

In general, produce with thicker skin that is peeled off, such as bananas and oranges, possesses lower concentrations of edible toxic residues.

I also encourage eating fruits and veggies raw, or at least increasing your consumption of raw, plant-based foods. Uncooked produce is higher in nutrients, antioxidants, repair enzymes, and water concentration, which all are key to minimizing signs of aging. (See Skin Commandment VI: Fight Free Radicals and Skin Commandment IV: Hydrate Holistically.)

Also, the process of heating and cooking foods introduces potential carcinogens, destroys nutrients, denatures enzymes, and dehydrates food. Another definite no-no is "well done" or burnt food that contains highly oxidative chemicals and carcinogens such as acrylamides, found in burnt toast, or polycylic aromatic hydrocarbons, found in burnt barbecue or smoked foods.

145

Speaking of barbecue, if you insist on eating meat or dairy products, I urge you to consider buying products made from animals that were not injected with growth hormones. As stated, with respect to dairy products, particularly skim milk and cheese, several studies have linked hormones in these products to acne. More and more groceries now offer hormone-free meats and dairy products, which are the legal standard in most nations in the European Union.

As stated, fish is a preferable source of protein, but not all fish are equally nutritious. You already know salmon is rich in omega-3 fatty acids, but did you know that wild-caught salmon is healthier for you than farmed salmon? Wild salmon are better fed (unlike farmed salmon, which are fed dried food pellets), they have not been given antibiotics, they have not been treated with artificial red/orange dyes to enhance their color, and they offer much higher levels of omega-3s.

The best option is wild sockeye salmon from Alaska, which has the most favorable omega-3 to omega-6 ratio and is very high in antioxidants. (See "Super Foods" in Skin Commandment VI: Fight Free Radicals.)

What about tilapia? Fans of tilapia are legion—U.S. tilapia consumption was estimated at 2.5 million tons in 2010—but fans of tilapia should know that farm-raised tilapia is also low in omega-3s and is not a great dietary option.

Does this mean all wild-caught fish are healthy?

No.

According to the National Institute of Environmental Health Sciences (a division of the National Institutes of Health), the Food and Drug Administration, and the Environmental Protection Agency, consuming large quantities of fish "increases a person's exposure to mercury."

All fish, even wild-caught fish, contain mercury, but some less than others. Black cod (also known as sablefish), sardines, salmon, and herring have low levels of mercury. Fish with medium levels of mercury include halibut, Chilean sea bass, tuna, and snapper. Large, predatory fish—including shark, swordfish, king mackerel, and tilefish—contain exceedingly high levels of mercury and should be avoided or eaten rarely.

THE IDEAL DIET—GLUTTONS BEWARE

Of all the fad diets, latest food tips, and dietary recommendations, the *only* diet that has been scientifically proven to extend life is caloric restriction. The less consumed, the longer the lifespan. So when it comes to dietary intake for all foods, a low-calorie diet is by far the most important aspect, and moderation is the key to longevity.

Eczema and Food Allergies

Six to 10 percent of children have atopic dermatitis, a common form of eczema that presents as red, cracked, and itchy skin. A recent five-year study showed that children with severe cases of this form of eczema "generally have a higher incidence of developing food allergies."

The American Academy of Dermatology now recommends that children under five with this form of eczema be evaluated for food allergies to milk, egg, peanut, wheat, and soy products.

Exercise
for Youthful Skin

Exercise keeps you flexible, keeps you fit, and keeps you toned.

Guess what?
Exercise keeps you looking young.

How? Exercise delivers more nourishing blood and oxygen to every organ in the body, including skin. Increased blood flow also leads to more rapid elimination of toxins and wastes by pumping lymph and other fluids out of the skin—and that's good.

When You're Hot . . .

Our bodies are programmed for thermoregulation, which is our ability to keep our body temperature within safe boundaries to avoid hypothermia (low body temperature), hyperthermia (high body temperature), heat stroke, or other dangerous conditions.

This isn't about adding an extra layer or slipping off a sweater.

When you exercise, your body heats up. Thermoregulation kicks in, and the increase in blood flow causes the capillaries under the skin to dilate, releasing heat. You start to sweat—the body's built-in evaporation system—which keeps you from overheating.

When you're cold, the blood vessels in your skin constrict to redistribute blood flow and effectively preserve internal heat.

Dr. T's Smooth Skin Stretches

Here are some simple stretches to keep you limber with an added bonus to help your skin stay smooth and silky.

Neck Stretches: After you cleanse your face each morning and evening, give your neck a relaxing stretch. Turn your neck to the left. Turn your neck to the right. Drop your chin to your chest and then gently turn your head from side to side. Repeat. Apply a small amount of moisturizer on your neck and gently knead your muscles while you stretch.

Shoulder Stretches: Hunched over a keyboard much of the day? Every couple of hours, stand up and lift your shoulders to your ears. Drop them slowly. Repeat four times. Now, one arm at a time, reach across your chest and over your opposite shoulder. Place your opposite hand over the elbow that is reaching to gently aid the stretch. Breathe deeply. Grab some moisturizer, smooth it on your arms, hands, and shoulders, gently massaging your skin and loosening your muscles. Now get back to work.

Back Stretches: When you step out of the shower, take a minute to warm up your back muscles. Slowly bend forward, stretching your fingers toward the floor. Slowly pull back up. Repeat. On the last stretch, make good use of your time folded in half by slathering body lotion on your legs. Gently work the lotion deep into your skin and leg muscles.

What does exercise get you?
Plenty.

Besides the anti-aging benefits, here are some other perks:

- increased muscular strength
- stamina
- enhanced bone density
- extra flexibility
- more restful sleep
- a sense of well-being
- stress relief

But don't overdo it. When it comes to exercise, enough is enough.

Exercise Restraint

Exercise-related skin problems can occur even when you follow a balanced workout schedule.

If you notice any of the following common problems, see your dermatologist right away to avoid pain or further infection that may lead to days lost at the gym.

- blisters on the hands or feet
- athlete's foot
- jock itch
- toenail fungus
- acne from improper hygiene or tight-fitting clothes
- pressure ulcers from cycling
- friction-induced rashes from lack of padding or cushioning

USE COMMON SENSE—stop any exercise-related skin problems before they get out of hand.

We all know somebody who puts in much too much time at the gym, risking stress, strain, and injury. These individuals may also experience a loss of facial fat, fat that is normally resistant to weight loss, giving them sunken cheeks and hollow faces—not a good look. (See Skin Commandment VIII: Fill 'er Up).

More serious effects of over-exercising can include an increased risk of stroke, heart rhythm abnormalities, and the loss of menstrual periods in women.

For most people, I recommend three to four hours per week of moderate-intensity cardiovascular exercise plus two to three hours per week of controlled weight-bearing activities. The Department of Health and Human Services advocates thirty minutes of physical activity of some sort every day.

My best advice about exercise is to choose something you like to do so you will actually do it. To boost your commitment, hire a trainer or make appointments with yourself, blocking out time on the calendar for working out.

Stressed-Out Skin

Just as your skin is a reflection of your physical health, your mental health also is on display on your skin. Stress actually can trigger many skin diseases.

Neurodermatitis, a chronic itchy rash due to stress, is caused by inflamed sensory nerves in the skin. People with neurodermatitis go to their doctors, literally and figuratively scratching their heads and wondering where the new itch came from. The underlying issue is never one of skin, but one of stress.

Every day, devote at least fifteen to twenty minutes to quiet, alone time for meditation and reflection—the keywords being quiet *and* alone, *with no TV, music, Internet, or other distractions. Ideally, you should meditate outdoors and take advantage of nature's calming effects, but any quiet place will do. Breathe slowly and deeply, filling and emptying your lungs to maximum and minimum capacity. Try to clear your mind of all thoughts and concerns. In these moments of solitude and peace you will find clarity and relief for all of your day-to-day troubles.*

No pill, other than a "chill pill," will cure the problem.

Hives, shingles, psoriasis, rosacea, and eczema are all skin disorders that may be triggered by stress. Some acne is due to stress. We've all experienced "stress pimples" the night before a huge test, a big day at work, or other major life event. Stress acne occurs when stress hormones are released during periods of stress, causing oil glands to enlarge, increasing oil production, and clogging pores.

Never underestimate the effects that stress can have on the body or on your skin. Periods of unrelieved stress can lead to physical symptoms that go way beyond skin disorders, including the following:

• headaches	• anxiety
• high blood pressure	• depression
• heart palpitations	• sleep deprivation

Stress also ages your skin and overall appearance. Otherwise, how else is it possible that of two thirty-five-year-old individuals with the same skin tone, same amount of sun damage, living in the same climate, one can look so much older than the other? Simple—one has a more strenuous life and lives in a stressful state of mind.

Stress is destructive mentally and physically. Stress has profound effects on health and, therefore, beauty. Taking control of your stress—"getting a grip"—is essential to any long-term skin-care or anti-aging program.

Get Some Rest

TIRED?

Almost half of Americans ages thirteen to sixty-four do not get enough sleep. Some scientists blame our addiction to technology, which allows us to shop online in our pajamas, post on Facebook, watch the news, or surf the web late into the night.

HOW MUCH SLEEP IS ENOUGH?

The National Institutes of Health recommends eight hours per night for adults. Teens need nine hours or more. When you skimp on sleep, you build up a "progressive sleep debt" (each night, you get further and further behind the recommended number of hours of restful sleep) and no, you can't catch up on the weekend. Even

---

Dark Circles, Puffy Eyes

Do you blame the dark circles under your eyes on late nights or lack of sleep?

Don't.

Those dark circles are a result of thinning skin, loss of elasticity, enlarged blood vessels, and genetics. Fillers (Skin Commandment VIII) or laser treatments (Skin Commandment IX) may help. No "miracle cream" actually works—yet.

Puffy eyes in the morning? That's normal.

Our tears protect us from bacteria and keep particles from accumulating in the eyes. When you lie down—especially if you sleep on your stomach—those tears build up and stagnate under the eyelids, giving them a puffy look.

Consider sleeping with a good pillow to elevate your head or gently icing your eyes for a few minutes in the morning. Ice can be followed up with gentle massage (see Dr. T's Lymphatic Drainage Tip for Puffy Skin on the next page). Severe cases of morning eye swelling should be evaluated by an ophthalmologist.

Dr. T's Lymphatic Drainage Tip for Puffy Skin

Exercise helps pump fluid out of the skin and back into the bloodstream. To reduce puffiness, try superficial lymphatic drainage of the face and eyes with an osteopathic technique known as effleurage. Effleurage manually moves stagnant lymph in the superficial skin layers along natural lymph drainage patterns and back into the bloodstream. For the face, gently rake your fingertips along the central brow out towards the temples. Continue the stroke down the temples, over the cheeks, and backwards along the jaw line towards the ears. Now stroke down the neck muscles toward the collar bone. Repeat three to five times.

For the eyes, gently rake your fingertips from the inner, lower eyelids outward toward the temples. Continue the stroke down the temples, over the cheeks, and down the neck. Repeat three to five times.

if you think you are fine, a lack of sleep exacts a toll on your skin via stress hormones and oxidative stress.

TEND TO YOUR SPIRITUALITY

Researchers in the field of positive psychology are examining the effects of strong religious beliefs on happiness and longevity. Experts at the Mayo Clinic suggest that individuals who consider themselves spiritual feel a sense of purpose, connect to the world, release control, and expand their support network.

Why?

It could be that spirituality leads to stress relief, a sense of increased well-being that comes when you believe that you are not alone.

Some scientists say that we possess "a natural inclination for religious belief," perhaps developed in our earliest days when sharing a belief system strengthened survival skills. Others dispute that. Still, belief in a higher power provides meaning and context for many individuals, deepening self-worth and enriching connections with others.

Spirituality is a personal thing. For some people, spirituality means worship according to the teachings of a specific religious denomination. For others, personal styles of prayer, meditation, yoga, or volunteer service define spirituality. Some people find evidence of a higher power in nature, or art, or family. My personal spiritual life is defined by the teachings and practice of Christianity and in medical missionary service.

All these practices can reduce stress, and they not only make us happier, but they also may lead to a longer life and slow the process of aging. Whatever other healthy methods you turn to in order to relieve stress, consider calming down by tuning into your spiritual life.

The Last Word
for *The Skin Commandments*

Good skin care is good health care, and vice versa. Caring for your skin will protect your health, and tending to your body, mind, and spirit will reward you with incredible, healthy, glowing skin regardless of your age.

Choosing skin-care treatments and products can be confusing, but if you've read the book, you now understand that it's imperative to protect yourself from the sun and stay out of tanning beds.

You have specific guidelines for choosing sunscreen, cleansing, hydrating, and exfoliating your skin. You also know why all these steps are an important investment in keeping your skin healthy and beautiful.

If you were unsure before, now you understand exactly why it's important to choose topical skin-care products that will protect your skin from damage brought about by oxidative stress.

You have learned that almost anything about your skin that bothers you can be improved with state-of-the-art treatments by a board-certified dermatologist. Whether you turn to peels, Botox, fillers, or laser treatments—within days (sometimes minutes) you can begin enjoying the skin you see yourself in or the skin you once had.

It's all here in *The Skin Commandments*, which serves to get the conversation started between you and your dermatologist. My hope is that the conversation will motivate you to commit to taking good care of your skin and health every day. Actuarial tables and genetics aside, none of us knows exactly how long we will get to live. That is the perfect argument for living healthy, looking your best, and feeling great.

One last bit of advice: _____

For healthy, beautiful skin, follow the **Skin Commandments I-X.**

Glossary

antioxidants—vitamins and nutrients that neutralize oxygen-free radicals

astringent—a substance that causes tissue to shrink or tighten; the active ingredient found in most facial toners

atopic dermatitis—a chronic skin disorder that presents as red, cracked, and itchy skin

basel cell carcinoma—the most common skin cancer

carcinoma—cancer

chemical peels—skin exfoliation treatments that use a chemical to remove outer layers of skin

cherry angiomas—round, red spots on the body due to enlarged blood vessels

collagen—a structural protein in the skin

contact dermatitis—skin inflammation from contact with an irritating substance

dehydration—loss of water and salts in the body

dermabrasion—an aggressive surgical scraping treatment for sun-damaged or scarred skin

dermatoheliosis—skin signs of aging due to sun damage; a.k.a. photo-aging

dermis—layer of skin below the epidermis

elasticity—springiness; rubber band–like quality

elastin—a protein responsible for the skin's elasticity

emollients—ingredients that soften and soothe skin

enzymes—complex proteins in the body that aid in normal chemical reactions

epidermis—top layer of skin

exfoliation—removing the top layer of dry skin cells

fractionated laser—a laser that uses microbeams of light to safely resurface the skin

glabellar lines—frown lines between the eyebrows

granulomas—disfiguring nodules that may form under the skin due to injection of foreign substances

humectants—ingredients that promote water retention in the outer skin layer

hyperthermia—high body temperature

hypothermia—low body temperature

laser resurfacing—a laser procedure that removes outer skin layers in order to smooth the skin surface

liposomes—a type of cellular membrane

melanin pigment—the pigment found in skin that accounts for skin tone; the body's natural sunscreen

melanocytes—skin cells that make melanin pigment

melanoma—a dangerous form of skin cancer due to cancerous melanocytes

melasma—a condition characterized by blotchy facial skin, most commonly due to hormones

microdermabrasion—a gentle, skin scraping treatment

neocollagenesis—formation of new collagen

neurodermatitis—a chronic itchy rash due to emotional stress

noncomedogenic—a product that will not clog your pores

oxidative damage—tissue damage caused by oxygen-free radicals

oxygen-free radicals—highly destructive, electrically charged oxygen molecules that form due to normal chemical reactions in the body, aging, sunlight, and other external factors

photo-aging—the aging process initiated by sunlight

phytonutrients—nutrients derived from plants

retinoids—chemical compounds derived from vitamin A used in medications and cosmetics

rhinophyma—a severe form of rosacea that causes a rhinocerous-like enlargement of the nose

rosacea—a chronic, genetic skin disease characterized by facial redness

sebum—the skin's natural oil

skin turgor—a skin pull test that helps assess internal hydration

spider veins—small dilated blood vessels near the surface of the skin

squamous cells—cancerous cells that form on the surface of the skin

stratum corneum—outermost layer of the epidermis, responsible for skin texture (dry or moist)

subcutaneous—beneath the skin

super foods—foods full of high-powered antioxidants, vitamins, and nutrients

thermoregulation—the body's ability to keep our temperature within safe boundaries